Race, Culture and Ethnicity in Secure Psychiatric Practice

Forensic Focus

This series, edited by Gwen Adshead, takes the currently crystallising field of Forensic Psychotherapy as its focal point, offering a forum for the presentation of theoretical and clinical issues. It will also embrace such influential neighbouring disciplines as language, law, literature, criminology, ethics and philosophy, as well as psychiatry and psychology, its established progenitors.

Also in the series:

Managing High Security Psychiatric Care
Edited by Charles Kaye and Alan Franey
ISBN 1 85302 581 X pb
ISBN 1 85302 582 8 hb
Forensic Focus 9

**Forensic Nursing and Multidisciplinary Care of
the Mentally Disordered Offender**
Edited by David Robinson and Alyson Kettles
ISBN 1 85302 754 5 pb
ISBN 1 85302 753 7 hb
Forensic Focus 14

**Forensic Psychotherapy
Crime, Psychodynamics and the Offender Patient**
Edited by Christopher Cordess and Murray Cox
ISBN 1 85302 634 4 pb
ISBN 1 85302 240 3 hb
Forensic Focus 1

A Practical Guide to Forensic Psychotherapy
Edited by Estela V. Welldon and Cleo Van Velsen
Forewords by Fiona Caldicott and Helena Kennedy
ISBN 1 85302 389 2 pb
Forensic Focus 3

**The Arts in Health Care
A Palette of Possibilities**
Edited by Charles Kaye and Tony Blee
ISBN 1 85302 360 4

Forensic Focus 13

Race, Culture and Ethnicity in Secure Psychiatric Practice
Working with Difference

Edited by Charles Kaye, Former Chief Executive,
Special Hospitals Service Authority
and Tony Lingiah, Broadmoor Hospital Authority

Jessica Kingsley Publishers
London and Philadelphia

First published in the United Kingdom in 2000 by
Jessica Kingsley Publishers Ltd
116 Pentonville Road,
London N1 9JB, England
and
325 Chestnut Street,
Philadelphia, PA19106, USA

www.jkp.com

Copyright © 2000 Jessica Kingsley Publishers

Library of Congress Cataloging in Publication Data
A CIP catalog record for this book is available from the Library of Congress

British Library Cataloguing in Publication Data
Race and culture in secure psychiatric practice: working with difference. – (Forensic focus; 13)
1. Psychiatry, Transcultural – Great Britain
I. Kaye, Charles   II. Lingiah, Tony
362.2'0941

ISBN 1 85302 696 4 pb
ISBN 1 85302 695 6 hb

Printed and Bound in Great Britain by
Athenaeum Press, Gateshead, Tyne and Wear

To the staff and patients
at Broadmoor Hospital

Whoever degrades another degrades me,
and whatever is done or said returns at last to me.

Walt Whitman
Song of Myself

Acknowledgements

The origins of this book lie in work undertaken under the auspices of Broadmoor Hospital. We are particularly grateful to Joanna Sheehan, then Acting Chief Executive of the Hospital, and Kelvin Cheatle, Director of Human Resources, for their support and encouragement. Dr Julie Hollyman has continued this support since becoming Chief Executive.

Dr Chandra Ghosh has been a constant advocate of the need for more education and understanding in the area of ethnic difference and we are both indebted to her for her enthusiasm and lively and helpful (if at times provocative) suggestions. She has been an inspiration.

Many other people have helped us in different ways and it is a pleasure to recognise their assistance:

Martin Butwell and Phil Connell, for help with statistics.

Veena Soni Raleigh, for permission to use the table on page 13

Mike Jones and Paul Robertson for permission to use photographs.

Les Martin, Dave Henry, Mandy Brough, John Clay, Ruth Preese and Elaine Elvey for help with finding illustrations.

Nizar Boga, David Usoro and Farzana for permission to use their artwork.

Anthony Roach for his poem quoted on page 197

Cathy Nightingale for her imaginative and sensitive work in designing the front and back covers.

Helen Wood for helpful suggestions.

Allison Farrar and Judy Phillips for their help at Broadmoor Hospital Library and Brenda Goddard and her team for help at the library of the Royal Hampshire County Hospital.

Our particular thanks go to Linda Lowe who has shepherded the manuscript through its many stages, showing patience and good humour throughout.

Charles Kaye and Tony Lingiah

Contents

PART I

Structures and Power

CHAPTER 1

Difference Described

Charles Kaye

Hapley, for I am black.

Othello

INTRODUCTION

This chapter draws a picture, both nationally in the UK and specifically within the National Health Service (NHS), of disadvantage for ethnic minorities. It presents briefly evidence illustrating aspects of such disadvantage over a range of social institutions. Finally it describes the current position with regard to both staff and patients in the Forensic Psychiatric Service.

NATIONAL CONTEXT

In most of the social institutions in the UK that are responsible for providing facilities, controlling behaviour or meeting need, there is evidence of problems arising from inequality and prejudice focused on minorities within the community. The minorities are usually immigrant groups, for instance from Ireland, the Indian subcontinent, the Caribbean or Africa, and the problems are a compound of the disadvantages clustering around low income and status and of disdain and resentment expressed (towards the 'newcomers') by many of the surrounding majority. The very institutions which struggle to meet the difficulties are themselves, since they are broadly of the majority, flawed by the prejudice they formally condemn.

While leaders, the law and official policies are firmly united in condemning prejudice and promoting equality, the practice of society and its institutions demonstrates repeatedly that discrimination against minorities is ingrained in our social fabric. The most cursory scrutiny of the media and journals will provide evidence of this and of the exasperatingly slow pace of change. The thick slit of prejudice remains in a stubborn layer and only requires the slightest agitation for it to colour the mainstream of our lives. The working of our national institutions abundantly illustrates this – as do the daily experiences of those from within the minorities. As the Scarman Report summarised the position, reflecting on inner city problems after the riots of the early 1980s:

> The core of the problem is this: a decaying urban structure, with its attendant evils of bad-quality and inadequate housing, and a lack of job opportunities, with its inevitable evil of high unemployment. These depressing conditions coexist with the crucial social fact that these areas have a high proportion of ethnic minority groups – blacks and Asians. And these groups believe and feel, with considerable justification, that it is the colour of their skins, and their first or second generation immigrant origins which count against them in their bid for a fair share of our society. (Scarman 1981)

In the brief overview that follows, the key aim is to illustrate the disadvantages that ethnic minorities face today in the UK and to draw out some of the consequences for individuals and society as a whole. The exploration of explanations behind the statistics and perceptions is deliberately not mapped here. Disadvantage has many facets: some arise from prejudice and resentment; some from comparative social and financial status; some from the time required for integration through individual effort. The common factor stressed is the reality of disadvantage.

Who are the minorities?

The main factor among minorities within the UK would seem to be immigration. Many comprise individuals and groups from other countries looking for life and a 'new start' in Britain. Sometimes this will be associated with asylum, or the escape from oppressive conditions in their own country; sometimes it is linked to the prospect of more opportunity in a new country. This is not a phenomenon confined to this country; it can be mirrored in the contemporary experience of a number of European neighbours and of the USA.

If the 1991 census is taken as a starting point, the largest minority are the Irish. That count showed that there were nearly 900,000 Irish-born people in Britain. 'If second and third generations are considered the number rises to over two million' (Health Education Authority (HEA) 1998a). There is a growing literature examining the inequalities suffered by this minority:

> There is now considerable evidence that all of the ethnic minorities in Britain, the Irish have the poorest record of both physical and mental health. (Bracken et al. 1998)

The link with other factors is also stressed:

The Irish in Britain are a stark example of the link between poor housing and ill health ... Mortality data since 1984 has shown high levels of premature mortality in Irish people in Britain and recent research shows this pattern persists into the second generation ... Irish people are significantly less likely to be owner occupiers and are more likely to be in local authority housing, the private rented sector or in overcrowded accommodation sharing amenities. (Tilki 1998, p.17)

In many respects Irish immigrants and their descendants are a hidden white minority whereas other groups are identified primarily by the colour of their skin.

The 1991 census data can be analysed in this context, as shown in Figure 1.1.

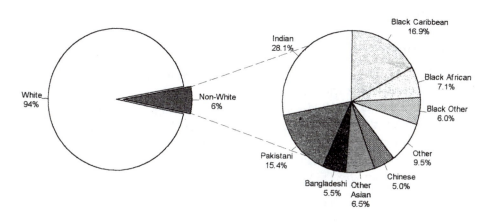

Figure 1.1 Ethnic composition of the population of England and Wales
Source: 1991 Census

The first wave of postwar immigration started with the arrival of 500 people from the Caribbean on the *SS Empire Windrush* at Tilbury Docks on 22 June 1948. Significantly now there are second and third generations from the original immigrants and it is estimated that, for instance, half of the African-Caribbean community within the UK are British born (HEA 1998b).

The black and Asian communities, both migrants and British-born, will be focused upon in the context of our key social institutions. For convenience the term 'black' will, on occasion, be used as shorthand to include both black and Asian communities. We need to remember that there are different realities and different experiences contained within these minorities:

Within the ethnic minority population there is an increasing disparity between the circumstances of specific groups. The findings suggest that the South Asian population contains both the most and the least successful of the ethnic minority groups that we have studied. At one extreme we have the African Asian and Indian populations. These groups have higher proportions of well-qualified people, have attained comparable (or better) job levels to whites, and have unemployment rates closest to those found among the white population. At the opposite end of the spectrum there are the Pakistanis and the Bangladeshis. They retain the largest proportion, even among young people, with no formal qualifications of any ethnic groups. They have substantially lower job levels than people of other origins, and consistently suffer the highest rates of unemployment.

The Afro-Caribbean population tend to fall into a position which is somewhere in between these two extremes. The Chinese appear to be in a similar position to the African Asians and the Indians. (Jones 1993)

A brief review of key institutions draws the following pictures.

Education

A number of studies have demonstrated that African-Caribbean children were more likely to be excluded from school than their white counterparts (Bourne, Bridges and Searle 1994). A more recent publication, analysing the official government statistics, confirms 'previous research findings that black boys and girls are four to six times more likely to be permanently excluded than their white counterparts' (Commission for Racial Equality 1997). That report also quotes from an OFSTED publication:

> On average, Caribbean young men…appear to be achieving considerably below their potential… A combination of gender and racial stereotypes may make it more difficult for young black men to avoid being caught up in cycles of increasingly severe criticism and control. (OFSTED 1996, quoted in CRE 1997)

In 1998 the Education Secretary, David Blunkett, was quoted as saying – when introducing news of £430 million to be spent on the teaching of minorities – that:

> If you are black or of Pakistani or Bangladeshi origins, your chance of gaining five good GCSEs is half that of white pupils. (*The Times* 13.11.98)

Housing

The government's Social Exclusion Unit (1998) makes the following observation on rough sleeping:

Proportions of rough sleepers from ethnic minorities are typically five per cent or less. But voluntary organisations report that there are disproportionately high numbers of people from ethnic minorities amongst the single homeless population who live in hostels.

In 1998 Shelter, the charity dealing specifically with the homeless and housing problems, published an analysis of its client enquiries in 1997/98. This showed that 12 per cent of their clients were black (twice the proportion of the population at large) and that three-quarters of them were homeless or in danger of becoming so (Diaz 1998).

In an analysis of housing tenure, Diaz (1998) makes the following observations:

> There is no uniform pattern of tenure among the minority ethnic population ...there are major disparities in tenure patterns between the White population and among minority ethnic groups. The most marked difference is the levels of owner occupation ... 82% of Indian and 76% of Pakistani households own their homes but few are in either social or private rented housing. Indian households have a higher level of home ownership than their White counterparts. For people of Black origin patterns are totally different, for example 52% of Black African households and 46% of Black Caribbeans, rely on the social rented sector.
>
> The fact that some minority groups, in particular Indian and Pakistani households, have a high level of owner occupation, does not always imply higher status of employment or a higher standard of living. For example a survey in Scotland found that, due to the lack of suitable alternative accommodation, minority ethnic households often felt forced into owner occupation.

Furthermore, location, always the key factor in housing, has its own significance:

> Comparison at the national level will inevitably find much greater differences between white and ethnic minority accommodation than would be found by local level analysis, since the ethnic minority population has traditionally been concentrated into inner-city areas associated with lower quality housing. (Jones 1993)

Employment

Minority ethnic groups are over-represented among the long-term unemployed. Youth unemployment is consistently high across all groups, but is higher for those of black origin. By 1996/97 the rate of unemployment for this group was 35 per cent compared with 14 per cent of white youth (Office for National Statistics 1998).

The disadvantages faced by minority ethnic groups in the job market can be seen by looking at the economic activity rates and unemployment patterns for the different groups. In 1991 the proportion of economically active men who were in full-time employment was highest among the white group (69%) and lowest among the Pakistani group (47%). Black African, Pakistani and Bangladeshi groups were in the worst position with male unemployment rates three times higher than their white counterparts (Housing Corporation 1996, quoted in Diaz 1998).

An analysis carried out by the Policy Studies Institute in 1993 (Jones 1993) showed that:

> There has been an important change in the distribution of ethnic minorities between job levels. The proportion of Chinese, African Asian, and Indian male employees having jobs in the top category (professional, managerial, employer) is now as high as for white men, or higher. As shown by the earlier surveys, the job levels of Indian men are more polarised that those of white men: there is still a higher proportion of Indians than of whites in semi-skilled and unskilled manual jobs, but about the same proportion of Indians and whites in the top category. The same applies to the Chinese, to a greater degree. Afro-Caribbean men, as before, tend to be concentrated in skilled manual jobs, while Pakistani and Bangladeshi men still tend to be at much lower job levels than white men.

Overall, Jones (1993) concluded:

> Even within job levels, Pakistani and Bangladeshi workers have substantially higher unemployment rates than other groups. This remains the case if we control for age group, qualification, or region of residence. In some cases, controlling for such factors makes the difference even greater. The case of Afro-Caribbean people is more complex. They tend to be in a position which falls somewhere between those of the whites, African Asians, Indians and Chinese on the one hand, and the Pakistanis and Bangladeshis on the other. The Afro-Caribbean population is the longest-established of all the major post-1945 settlement groups included in this study.
>
> Their continuing position of overall disadvantage compared to the white population, and to groups within the more recently-arrived South Asian population, is therefore particularly striking.

Civil Service

"'The Civil Service must be part of, not apart from, the society it serves.'

Are you the person to make this happen? Can you spearhead efforts to improve the number and profile of people from ethnic minority backgrounds in the Civil Service?"

Cabinet Office advertisement *Observer* 12.9.99

The government's own figures show that at 1 April 1997, 5.7 per cent of non-industrial civil servants were of ethnic minority origin. (These figures derive from the response to a voluntary self-classification questionnaire). Spread across different grades, the figures form the familiar pyramid: at the lowest grades, ethnic minorities make up 7.3 per cent of those replying; at the highest level, only 1.6 per cent (Government Statistical Service 1998).

A report on recruitment to the 'fast stream' schemes in the Civil Service in 1997/98 showed that only 7 black or Asian graduates were among the total of 277 recruited. The success rate for ethnic minority candidates was 0.5 per cent compared with 3.1 per cent for whites. In the general (i.e. Whitehall Central Government) departments no minority candidates at all were recruited in that year (*Public Service Magazine* Dec/Jan 1998/99).

Criminal justice system

The broad contours of the historical processes of criminalisation of migrant communities are now relatively uncontroversial, whether the group concerned is the Irish at the turn of the century, Maltese and Cypriots in the 1930's and 1940's, or the British black community over the last 30 or more years. Racist stereotypes of racial difference feed into public knowledge and policing practice. A conflict with the reality of 'unjust' policing echoes through the 'due process of the law' into courts and penal institutions, reinforcing the portrayal of migrant groups as involved in putatively specific forms of criminal activity and legitimising particular repressive policing strategies targeted on those communities. The potential for the perpetuation of this pattern is exacerbated by the institutionalisation of stereotypes in the fabric of the agencies of social reproduction. (Keith 1993)

Police

The problems in terms of the relationship between police forces and ethnic minorities have been well publicised. This particularly sensitive area, where enforcing and control are key activities and where 'zero tolerance' is a term of approval, is an incubator where prejudices and misunderstanding flourish. Ethnic minorities are under-represented in police forces: 2 per cent nationally; 3 per cent in London where over a fifth of the population is from ethnic minorities; 4.4 per cent in Leicestershire – the highest percentage in the country – where the minority groups are 11 per cent of the population (*The Times* 20.10.98).

The requirement for all police forces to monitor stop/searches which was first introduced in 1993 did not originally ask them to differentiate between the groups in the 'ethnic minority' category but the published figures have consistently shown that, overall, ethnic minorities are stopped and searched more frequently than whites – although the pattern varies considerably between forces. The Metropolitan police area has the greatest number of searches and the highest ethnic minority population. The 1996/97 figures show for the Metropolitan Police:

> an overall ratio of 2.5 ethnic minority stops to one of a white person; but this figure 'unpacked' to a figure of 4.4 stops of black people and 1.2 for stops of Asians. In Leicestershire similarly the semblance of parity in the HMIC returns masked a search rate for black people which was more than five times the rate for whites. (Fitzgerald and Sibbitt 1997, p.40)

A 1998 study, *Deaths in Police Custody* (Leight, Johnson and Ingram 1998) which examines the circumstances of 277 deaths during 1990–96 found that the percentage of black detainees whose deaths were linked to police actions was significantly higher than deaths of whites. For 17 of these deaths, ethnicity data were not available, but of the remaining 260, the Home Office study found that 226 detainees were white, 19 black and 15 of Asian or other ethnic background. It found that nine – 47 per cent – black detainees had died in circumstances associated with police action or in accidents where officers were present. By contrast only 16 – 7 per cent – white detainees died in similar circumstances:

> The question of 'over-representation' has been at the heart of the 'race and crime' debate. Specifically, the accumulated evidence and statistics have shown black people to be over-represented in criminal justice figures relative to their presence in the population at large; and interpretations of this have spanned two poles – from inference of large-scale discrimination on the one hand to assumptions about black criminality on the other. (Fitzgerald and Sibbitt 1997, p.90)

At the end of 1998 Dan Crompton, Inspector of Constabulary, was quoted as saying with regard to race relations policing:

> There are pockets of good practice but generally there is room for substantial improvement. (*The Times* 19.12.98)

Prisons

The Home Office's annual report on prison statistics (Home Office 1998) offers the following information:

- On 30 June 1997, 11,200 people in Prison Service establishments in England and Wales belonged to ethnic minority groups. This was 10 per cent more than the 10,200 held in June 1996 but the rate of increase was slightly less than the 11 per cent rise between 1996 and 1997 for the prison population generally.
- Ethnic minority groups made up 18 per cent of the male and 25 per cent of the female prison populations at the end of June 1997.
- Greater proportions of male white prisoners were in prison for violent or sexual offences (31%) or for burglary (19%) than black prisoners

(25% and 11% respectively). Black male sentenced prisoners were more likely than white males to be held for robbery (24% compared with 12%) or drug offences (21% compared with 12%).

- In mid-1997 16 per cent of the black sentenced adult male population were serving sentences of over 4 years. This compares with 47 per cent for white sentenced adult males, 59 per cent of sentenced adult male South Asians, and 61 per cent of sentenced adult males from Chinese and other ethnic groups.
- The incarceration rate for whites ... is 176 per 100,000 population. This compares with 1249 for members of black groups and 150 for members of South Asian groups.

The courts

The evidence is that black defendants see magistrates' courts as police courts.

Courtney Griffiths, QC, Society of Black Lawyers, *The Times* 21.11.98

In her study for The Royal Commission on Criminal Justice, Marion Fitzgerald (1993) drew a number of significant conclusions:

There is considerable evidence that Afro-Caribbeans are more likely not to admit to the offences of which they are accused. At the outset, this draws them more deeply into the criminal justice process and makes it more likely that they will be convicted earlier in their criminal careers since it renders them ineligible to be cautioned and more likely, instead, to be charged. Studies of cautioning do, indeed, show that rates are lower for Afro-Caribbeans, and that the differences may be accounted for by differences in admissions of guilt which have further implications at the sentencing stage. (p.5)

And further:

The research available addressed many of the central concerns which have been raised by ethnic minorities about their experience of criminal justice. It does not do so definitively, however, and many gaps remain. Yet Hood adds weight to the evidence already accumulated which strongly suggests that, even where differences in social and legal factors are taken into account, there are ethnic differences in outcomes which can only be explained in terms of discrimination. And he raises the further possibility that apparently legitimate 'legal' considerations (in particular the higher penalties associated with 'not guilty' pleas) may themselves constitute indirect discrimination. (p.31)

At the end of her examination, she concludes:

In sum, the evidence presented here suggests that two propositions need constantly to be borne in mind when considering the relevance of any aspects of the criminal justice process to ethnic minorities: (p.38)

- The workings of the system generally are characterised by considerable variation; and the impact of these variations may fall unevenly on different ethnic groups.
- The decisions of criminal justice agencies (and other relevant bodies, including the legal profession and forensic 'experts') interact with and compound each other. None can be viewed in isolation; for if there are even small ethnic differences in the key decisions taken by each, their cumulative impact may be very large indeed. (Fitzgerald 1993)

Summary

This brief examination does not pretend to be a full study of any of the institutions considered. The studies cited are only indicators and their detailed interpretation requires further attention. It is also acknowledged that in each service or institution there is a commitment to equality and fairness and an official deprecation of situations where that standard is not achieved. However, the practical evidence consistently shows unexplained gaps between intention and action, between policy and results. There is an overall indication that on a wide front in our social fabric it can be a disadvantage to be from an ethnic minority group.

These vignettes demonstrate that organisations, on a vertical internal basis, are unable consistently to operate fairly and with equity. When it comes to the horizontal links, say to the lifetime experience of a young black male being shuttled between many (or all) of these services, the picture is even more disturbing. The cumulative effects of black disadvantage vividly illustrate how far we have to go.

THE NATIONAL HEALTH SERVICE

A Sandwell Healthcare NHS Trust Hospital has offered to remove 'negro' from a pre-operation form after a black patient complained that it was offensive.

The Times 2.9.99

The Chairman of the Commission for Racial Equality, Herman Ouseley, reviewed progress towards equality in the NHS thus:

Until we combine these three elements – leadership by everyone in a position of responsibility; effective, accountable and measured management of performance; and pressure from those for whom equality outcomes are still not being delivered – then progress in the NHS will be very patchy and in some areas non-existent. (Ouseley 1998, p.18)

Any analysis, however brief, must look at the two dimensions of the issue within the service: equality in matters of treatment and care, and equality in terms of staffing and opportunity.

Staffing

National statistics on NHS staff include a breakdown by ethnic origins. For all non-medical staff (as at 30.9.97):

> 89.9% were white
>
> 3.1% were black
>
> 1.5% were Asian
>
> 1.8% were other
>
> 3.7% were unknown

These figures are qualified with the rider: 'Figures should be treated with caution as they are based on the 68% of Hospital and Community Health Service organisations that reported 90% or more valid ethnic codes' (Department of Health 1998a).

No analysis is offered of ethnicity of staff in terms of age groups or managerial position. Anecdotal comment suggests that ethnic minorities are significantly under-represented in senior management grades.

A report in the *Journal of Health Management* (May 1998) quoted the findings of a study by Stephen Pudney and Michael Shields of Leicester University that 'men are consistently promoted faster than women, while white nurses of both sexes advance more quickly than black or Asian nurses.'

The position with regard to medical and dental staff (as at 30.9.97) is reported by the Department of Health (1998b) as (note that figures quoted in the publication only add to 99%):

> 82% were white
>
> 1% were black
>
> 5% were Indian/Pakistani/Bangladeshi
>
> 1% were Chinese
>
> 4% were other
>
> 6% were unknown (not stated)

Analysed by grade the picture is as shown in Table 1.1.

Table 1.1 EEA qualified staff by ethnic origin (percentages)

	Not stated	White	Non-white
All staff	6	82	12
Consultant	6	89	5
Associate specialist	6	84	10
Staff grade	6	80	14
Registrar group	5	81	14
Senior House Officer	6	74	20
House Officer	6	72	23
Other hospital staff	8	85	7

The more junior the grade, the higher the percentage of ethnic minorities.

An examination of Distinction awards to consultants in terms of their ethnic background suggested that while 13.9 per cent of all consultants came from ethnic minorities only 6.2 per cent of awards went to those from such minority backgrounds (Esmail et al. 1998).

A study carried out in 1995 suggested that white candidates were four times more likely to be accepted in some hospital medical schools than ethnic minority candidates (Esmail et al. 1995). Other studies have suggested possible discrimination in the work of the General Medical Council (Esmail and Everington 1994) and discrimination in shortlisting practices (Esmail and Everington 1993, 1997).

Forensic Psychiatric Service

The Forensic Psychiatric Service marks the area on the map of the country's public service where the law and psychiatry intersect. The question of determining responsibility for an individual's aberrant behaviour, of distinguishing between 'bad' and 'mad', is at the centre of this part of the NHS. The identification of, and treatment and care for, mentally disordered offenders is a difficult and controversial process where society's ambivalence and psychiatry's limitations make a clinical judgement a high-risk zone for all concerned. A full exposition of these issues can be found in Kaye and Franey (1998, Chapter 1).

It may be regarded as something of a misnomer to describe the specialist provision as a 'service'. There is a national (England and Wales) tertiary supra-regional facility provided in three large psychiatric hospitals (Ashworth,

Broadmoor and Rampton). They are managed in conditions of strict security to treat and detain patients with a serious mental disorder and a history of, or propensity towards, violent behaviour: 'Across the three hospitals nearly one-third of residents have killed, around 10% committed a sexual offence, about 10% arson and almost everyone else non-fatal but serious personal violence' (Taylor *et al.* 1998).

These hospitals are linked to a network of 'medium secure units' which provide a complementary service of a lower degree of security for individuals considered to be less dangerous. These units are smaller, up to 100 beds but generally around 40–50 beds. They usually include community and 'outreach' services.

In addition there is a significant, and increasing, private sector provision of medium secure services which grows according to demand and entrepreneurial ambition. There is also an important link with the population in prisons where the extensive incidence of mental illness has been well documented (Gunn, Maden and Swinton 1991).

Although all these services focus on a relatively small population of patients (totalling probably less than 10,000), there is limited cohesion between the constituent parts despite major organisational reforms in 1989 and 1996. A further reform is currently being planned to attempt to improve working together.

The close relationship between the criminal justice service and the forensic psychiatric service is underlined by shared problems relating to black and ethnic minorities.

Across this part of the NHS it is difficult to gather figures relating to staff and their origins since the service is provided within many different Trusts. However, figures are available for the three Special Hospitals (as at 13 October 1997), a shown in Table 1.2.

Table 1.2 Staff ethnicity profile for the three special hospitals

	White	%	Black	%	Indian/ Pakistani	%	Chi nese	%	Other/ Not known	%
Nursing qualified	1133	91.44	25	2.01	6	0.48	3	0.24	72	5.81
Nursing unqualified	1016	95.13	5	0.47	2	0.18	–	0.00	45	4.21
A&C	401	96.39	2	0.48	1	0.24	–	0.00	12	2.88
Ancillary	443	96.72	3	0.66	1	0.22	–	0.00	11	2.40
Rehab/ O.T.s	143	92.86	–	0.00	1	0.65	–	0.00	10	6.49
P.A.M.S.	191	96.46	–	0.00	–	0.00	–	0.00	7	3.54
Maintenance & Engineering	39	100.00	–	0.00	–	0.00	–	0.00	–	0.00
Social Work, Psychology Lecturers	119	92.25	–	0.00	2	1.55	–	0.00	8	6.20
Medical	54	58.06	2	2.15	14	15.05	–	0.00	23	24.73
Managers	183	95.31	–	0.00	1	0.52	–	0.00	8	4.17
TOTAL	3722	93.38	37	0.94	28	0.71	3	0.08	196	4.92

Source: High Security Psychiatric Services Commissioning Board

On analysis this shows a total of less than 2 per cent of staff coming from black or Asian backgrounds; 41 nurses from such backgrounds out of a total of 2149. Only within the medical staff were such minorities significantly represented (17.2%). The numbers are much lower than national figures and minorities are not represented at senior levels, with the exception of the consultant grade. This picture is particularly significant when the patient population's ethnic origins are analysed.

Interesting figures are available from Broadmoor Hospital which track the progress with regard to the recruitment and retention of staff from ethnic minorities (Table 1.3).

	Starters			Leavers		
	White	Black/Asian	Others/ unknown	White	Black/Asian	Others/ unknown
1994/95	84	3	5	138	10	4
1995/96	72	4	5	185	3	8
1996/97	94	8	3	134	13	3
1997/98	127	17	11	175	8	3

Table 1.3 Broadmoor Hospital: staff turnover by ethnic group 1994–98

Source: Broadmoor Hospital Personnel Department

Over the four-year period the numbers of ethnic minorities joining (32) and those leaving (34) more or less balance out. However, the most recent year (1997/98) shows by far the largest number (17) of recruits.

Morbidity and treatment

There is a growing literature examining the morbidity and mortality figures for different ethnic groups and many attempts to explain the differences which are revealed (e.g. Drever and Whitehead 1997; Nazroo 1997; Raleigh, Kiri and Balarajan 1996). There has also been examination of the disadvantaged positions that minorities may occupy with regard to accessing health services and treatment (Balajaran and Raleigh 1993a; Begum 1995; McIver 1994; Nazroo 1997).

With psychiatry, and forensic psychiatry in particular, such differences and discrepancies carry different connotations and significance. Chapters 3 and 4 of this book consider the sometimes uneasy relationship between prevailing social values and the practice of psychiatry. Those analyses give some indications of the complex networks that link society, its ethnic minorities, crime and mental illness. There are statistical summaries which, at the very least, are statements asking difficult questions.

In 1992 the Department of Health and Home Office reported that:

Black people who come to the attention of psychiatric services are more likely to be:

- removed by the police to place of safety under Section 136 of the Mental Health Act 1983

- detained in hospital under Sections 2, 3 and 4 of the Act

- diagnosed as suffering from schizophrenia or other forms of psychotic illness

- detained in locked wards of psychiatric hospitals
- given higher dosages of medication.

They are also less likely than white people to:

- receive appropriate and acceptable diagnosis or treatment at an early stage
- receive treatments such as psychotherapy or counselling.

Furthermore:

- 16% of Section 136 requests for approved social workers involved non-white people (10% Afro-Caribbean) compared with 6.4% in the study population;
  - the average referral rate per 100,000 population was 116.7
  - the average referral rate per 100,000 of the Asian population was 54.3
  - the average referral rate per 100,000 of the Afro-Caribbean population was 204 (Barnes and Maples 1990);
- the detention rate for the first generation male Afro-Caribbeans is five times as high as for whites and for second generation male Afro-Caribbeans it is nine times as high. (Department of Health and Home Office 1992a)

More recently a five-year prospective study (Goater *et al.* 1999) found that:

Our data confirm the excess of schizophrenia and non affective psychosis in black people living in the UK.

And that:

Something 'goes wrong' for black people relative to others later in the illness and this deterioration occurs despite the similar nature of the illness and frequency of service contact in all ethnic groups.

The Mental Health Act Commission, in their *Eighth Biennial Report* (1999), detailed the results of a survey that they had asked hospitals to carry out:

Hospitals were asked to record the number of patients who had been made subject to a section of the Mental Health Act during 1996/97 and 1997/98.

After tabulating the results (covering over 29,000 admissions in 1996/97 and over 33,000 in 1997/98) they warn that the outcome must be treated with caution. At best, they say, it gives an indication of trends. But these trends suggest that:

The use of the Act for black ethnic groups is over six times greater than the proportion of such groups in the population, while the use for Asian groups is roughly in line with the (1991) census.

Special hospitals

The in-patient population of the special hospitals analysed in terms of ethnic origin is shown in Table 1.4.

	Male		Female		Total
	Non-white	Total	Non-white	Total	
1988	198	1385	33	349	1734
1989	214	1385	30	330	1715
1990	218	1374	28	317	1691
1991	223	1387	28	298	1685
1992	224	1373	28	284	1657
1993	226	1338	26	258	1596
1994	221	1269	27	248	1517
1995	236	1256	29	232	1488
1996	240	1233	32	226	1459
1997	237	1201	29	222	1423

Table 1.4 Gender and ethnicity 1988–97: in-patient population totals for all special hospitals

Source: Statistical Service, Professorial Unit, Broadmoor Hospital

Thus for men, while the overall patient population has declined over the decade from nearly 1400 to 1200, the ethnic minority percentage has increased: in 1988 they represented 14.3 per cent of the population; in 1997, 20 per cent. For women, the overall population has been reduced by over a third while the number from ethnic minorities has remained very similar: 33 (9.4%) in 1988, 29 (13%) in 1997.

Figures for patient numbers in other parts of the forensic service are not easily obtainable. The annual summary of patients formally detained has no information about ethnic origins: this information is apparently not gathered centrally (Department of Health 1998c). This is an omission which needs to be made good. Anecdotally it would appear that forensic units closely linked to major urban centres have significant numbers of black patients, usually African-Caribbean. An analysis of admissions to one London-based service (Mohan *et al.* 1997) showed that 37 per cent of first admissions during the period 1983–95 were African-Caribbeans. An accurate and cumulative record nationally is a necessary piece of information to identify trends and increase awareness. If the special hospital picture is replicated in other elements of the forensic psychiatric service, there is a problem nationwide. We are no longer talking about a migrant population newly arrived; admissions are regularly British born, second generation.

Leaving causes to one side, let us look at consequences. One can anticipate some of the practical problems which arise when a predominantly white staff is caring for a significant black minority whose experience of social institutions is characteristically negative and who now find themselves being detained for the purpose of treatment.

An articulate and radical view of such a situation is put by Sonia Stephen, a psychotherapist:

> All institutions that have a European foundation are bad for black people, as our role within them is to be recipients of negative projections. Mental health institution are just places that large numbers of us will go through as we struggle to adapt to unnatural and unspiritual ways of living that are not of our making. (Stephen 1997)

In a different vein and using language of equal conviction, if less passion, the Blackwood Inquiry team observed of Broadmoor Hospital:

> We have described previously a culture within the hospital that is based on white European norms and expectations. As such, there exists a subtle, unconscious on the whole, but nevertheless effective form of organisational racism. Decisions on the treatment and management of patients are often influenced by this subliminal racism, where preconceived stereotypes play as great a part as individual needs. Racism is not simply the use of racist language; it can be far more subtle.
>
> Staff and management at Broadmoor Hospital do not seem to appreciate how this subtle form of racism operates and the part it plays in everyday decisions. It is not enough to proclaim that all patients are treated the same; that is not equality. It tends to erode ethnic differences and to discriminate most against the most different. In order to ensure all patients receive equal treatment senior management need to show a clear commitment to eliminating racism in all its forms. (Prins et al. 1993)

Those responsible for providing a service cannot reshape society and its treatment of ethnic minorities but they do have a duty to ensure that fair and equal treatment is offered to patients in their care. This is no easy task given the accumulation of prejudice and resentment that clearly exists.

CHAPTER 2

Mental Health in Black and Ethnic Minorities

An Epidemiological Perspective

Veena Soni Raleigh

INTRODUCTION

Black and ethnic minority people in Britain who are mentally ill suffer the double discrimination frequently associated with mental illness and race. Issues relating to race and culture in mental health services are causing increasing concern among ethnic minority communities and healthcare providers. There is much speculation and controversy about the levels and causes of mental illness experienced. There are concerns about over-diagnosis and over-representation in acute care for some ethnic groups, and about under-diagnosis, under-utilisation and unmet need in others. It is widely believed that mainstream mental health services often fail to meet ethnic minority needs. Racism in mental health care is a frequent theme in the literature, predominating to a much greater extent than in other literature on ethnic minority health.

If the goal of equity in quality mental health care provision for all is to be realised, epidemiological monitoring of need, access to care, and outcomes is vital. This chapter reviews the epidemiological literature on race and mental health. It is based on published literature, although much of the experience of black and ethnic minority people who are mentally ill, carers, providers and the communities at large, is unresearched and undocumented. The findings of published research are often challenged, both on methodological grounds and on more fundamental questions about the relevance of Eurocentric diagnostic categories and interpretations. Non-availability of data and limitations of available data seriously constrain the scope of analysis.

The term black and ethnic minority is used here to refer to people of Asian (Indian, Pakistani, Bangladeshi), Caribbean and African origin, the largest non-white minority groups in Britain. Although other ethnic minority populations (including white minorities such as the Irish) also have distinctive health experiences, they are not discussed here because of restricted space.

ENGLAND'S BLACK AND ETHNIC MINORITY COMMUNITIES

England is a multiracial country with 3 million non-white people, constituting 6 per cent of the total population (1991 Census). Indians form the largest group; next come the Caribbeans and Pakistanis, followed by Africans, Bangladeshi and the Chinese (See Figure 1.1, p.13). There are numerous smaller groups, e.g. Vietnamese, Turks, and people from Sri Lanka and the Middle East. The geographical distribution across the country varies between the different ethnic groups (Balarajan and Raleigh 1992).

The strong association between socio-economic deprivation and mental illness is well established, although the cause and effect process works both ways (Dohrenwend et al. 1992). Deprivation, unemployment, poor housing, and social isolation can contribute to mental illness (social causation). The causal process can also work in the opposite direction, that is, severe mental illness such as schizophrenia can cause sufferers to become socially isolated, unemployed and homeless (social selection).

Most ethnic minority communities experience greater socio-economic deprivation than the majority population, with higher unemployment (Figure 3.1), lower home ownership (Figure 3.2), and lower levels of tertiary education (Figure 3.3). They also experience more chronic illness (Figure 3.4), and are disproportionately represented in low-paid work, poor housing, and high-crime inner city areas. There are marked differences in household composition, with higher proportions of African-Caribbeans in single-person and single-parent households, and higher proportions of Asians in extended family households (Figure 3.5). All these factors influence mental health. Compared with the general population, higher proportions of ethnic minority people believe that their health is adversely affected by socio-economic disadvantage (Health Education Authority 1994). The experience of racism compounds these effects, and adversely affects the outcome of those who become mentally ill.

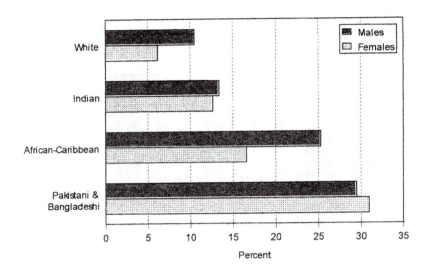

Figure 3.1 Unemployed (ages 16+), as a percentage of the economically active population, England and Wales

(Source: 1991 Census)

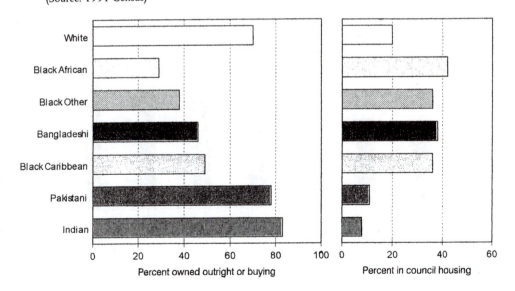

Figure 3.2 Housing tenure, England and Wales

(Source: 1991 Census)

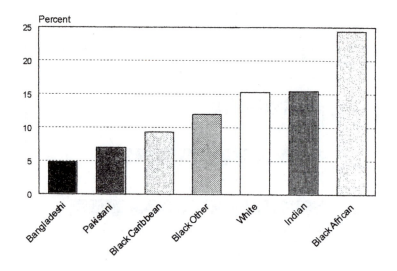

Figure 3.3 Percentage of people aged 18 years to pensionable ages qualified to diploma level or above, England and Wales

(Source: 1991 Census)

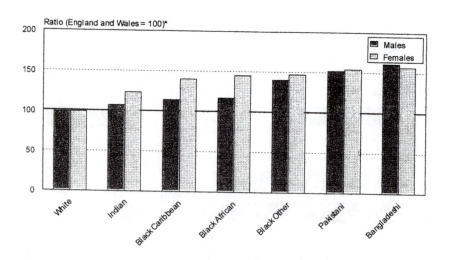

Figure 3.4 Age-standardised limiting long-term illness ratios, England and Wales. A ratio greater than 100 indicates a higher rate than the general population; a ratio less than 100 indicates a lower rate

(Source: 1991 Census)

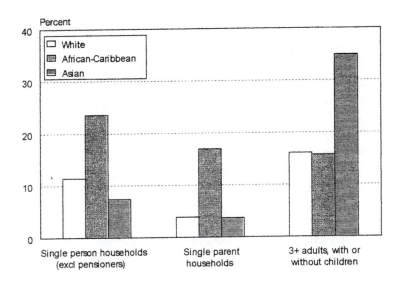

Figure 3.5 Percentage household composition, England and Wales
(Source: 1991 Census)

AFRICAN-CARIBBEAN PEOPLE
Prevalence of mental illness

The single most consistently reported finding from research into mental illness among ethnic minorities over three decades is the high rate of psychotic illness, schizophrenia in particular, in African-Caribbeans (Bebbington, Hurry and Tennant 1981; Bhugra *et al.* 1997; Bhui *et al.* 1998a; Birchwood *et al.* 1992; Carpenter and Brockington 1980; Cochrane 1977; Cochrane and Bal 1989; Commander *et al.* 1997; Cope 1989; Crowley and Simmons 1992; Dean, Downing and Shelley 1981; Dunn and Fahy 1990; Glover 1991; Harrison *et al.* 1988; Hutchinson *et al.* 1996; King *et al.* 1994; Koffman *et al.* 1997; Littlewood and Lipsedge 1988; McCreadie *et al.* 1997; McGovern and Cope 1987a; 1987b; Meltzer, Gill and Petticrew 1994; Nazroo 1997; Office for National Statistics 1995; Parkman *et al.* 1997; Sugarman and Craufurd 1994; Thomas *et al.* 1993; Van Os *et al.* 1996a, 1996b; Wessely *et al.* 1991). Schizophrenia is diagnosed 2–6 times more often in African- Caribbeans than in whites (Figure 3.6), with particularly high rates in young, UK-born men, who are more likely than other ethnic groups to be single, unemployed and living alone (Bhugra *et al.* 1997; Birchwood *et al.* 1992; Glover 1991; Harrison *et al.* 1988, Harvey *et al.* 1990; King *et al.* 1994; Littlewood and Lipsedge 1988;

McGovern and Cope 1987b, 1991; Owens, Harrison and Boot 1991; Thomas *et al.* 1993; Wessely *et al.* 1991). Excess risk is noted also by studies of familial risk, which show that siblings of second generation African-Caribbeans with schizophrenia have a significantly higher morbid risk of the illness than siblings of white counterparts (Hutchinson *et al.* 1996; Sugarman and Craufurd 1994). As no ethnic differences in parental morbid risks were noted, the studies concluded that there was a strong possibility of second generation vulnerability to selective environmental factors.

In contrast, the PSI survey found elevated rates of psychosis in Caribbean women but not Caribbean men (Nazroo 1997). It concluded that the overall excess was small and not statistically significant, although it identified a number of confounders which could bias the results. In particular, the survey did not cover institutions such as prisons and psychiatric hospitals. This would not introduce bias if all ethnic groups stood an equal risk of institutionalisation. However, the research to date shows without exception that African-Caribbeans (particularly young men) with a diagnosis of psychosis are highly over-represented in such institutions, and that the 'filters' between community and hospital/prison are less effective for them than for whites, making institutionalisation more likely (see sections on 'Pathways to Care' and 'Outcomes'). Recent studies of prison (Bhui *et al.* 1998a) and psychiatric hospitals in

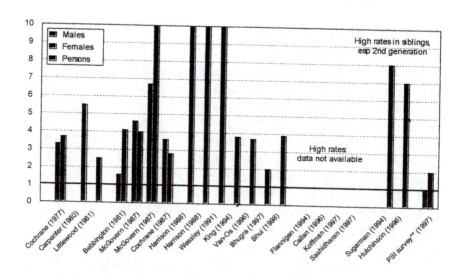

Figure 3.6 Schizophrenia among African-Caribbean people, England. A relative risk greater than 1 indicates a higher rate than the white population; a relative risk less than 1 indicates a lower rate

Thames Region (Koffman *et al.* 1997) and Birmingham (Commander *et al.* 1997) provide confirmation. Since psychotic illness invariably involves institutionalisation at some stage, if one ethnic group is more likely than another to be institutionalised, prevalence for that group will be underestimated in a community-based survey.

Non-psychotic disorders such as anxiety, depression, and alcohol abuse are often associated with socio-economic deprivation. Although African-Caribbeans are among the most deprived of Britain's ethnic minorities, several studies suggest that rates of minor psychiatric disorder are similar to or lower than in the white population (Bebbington *et al.* 1981; Cochrane 1977; Cochrane and Bal 1987; Dean, Downing and Shelley 1981; Gillam *et al.* 1989; Li, Jones and Richards 1994; Lloyd 1992, 1993; McKeigue and Karmi 1993; Owens, Harrison and Boot 1991; Thomas *et al.* 1993, 1989). Two national surveys, however, provide a measure of population-based psychiatric morbidity. Although the small numbers of non-whites in the ONS survey of psychiatric morbidity constrain the examination of ethnic differences, the survey reported a statistically significant excess of depression in African-Caribbean adults and an excess of psychoses in African-Caribbean women (Office for National Statistics 1995). The PSI survey of ethnic minorities likewise found higher rates of depression in Caribbeans (Nazroo 1997).

Explanations for high rates of schizophrenia

Various explanations have been advanced for the excess schizophrenia diagnosed in African-Caribbeans, although it is not clear why the arguments do not also apply to other ethnic minority groups. The explanations cannot be detailed here, but can be broadly summarised as follows:

- *Factors associated with the patient and his/her environment.* These include underlying biological or environmental susceptibility, e.g. the possibility of intra-uterine viral infection (Eagles 1991, 1992; Glover *et al.* 1994; Gupta 1993; O'Callaghan *et al.* 1991; Owen, Lewis and Murray 1988; *The Times* 13.04.95; Wessely *et al.* 1991) and environmental factors affecting the second generation (Bhugra *et al.* 1997; Hutchinson *et al.* 1996; Sugarman and Craufurd 1994; Takei *et al.* 1998); the effects of social adversity and racism (Bhugra *et al.* 1997; Burke 1984; Bowl and Barnes 1990; King *et al.* 1994; Lipsedge 1993; Littlewood and Lipsedge 1988; McKenzie *et al.* 1995; McGovern and Cope 1987b; Sashidharan 1993; Wessely *et al.* 1991); and the stress entailed in the migration process (Carpenter and Brockington 1980; Cochrane and Bal 1987; King *et al.* 1994; Littlewood and Lipsedge 1981).

- *Factors associated with psychiatric services and the criminal justice system.* The explanations range from relatively benign diagnostic incompetence through to the more serious charge of institutional racism, which enables psychiatric services and the criminal justice system to be used as instruments of social control over black and minority ethnic people (Cochrane and Bal 1987; Commission for Racial Equality 1995a; Department of Health and Home Office 1992a; Fernando 1988, 1991; Francis *et al.* 1989; Knowles 1991; Littlewood 1992b Littlewood and Lipsedge 1981, 1989; McGovern and Cope 1987b; Mercer 1984; Sashidharan and Francis 1993). It is said that the underlying factors are attributed to the racist historical origins of Western psychiatry and the Eurocentric diagnostic criteria used by a white establishment (Fernando 1991; Sashidharan 1993).

- *Flawed statistics/research (e.g. population denominators, diagnostic criteria and bias, hospital-based data).* However, numerous scientifically conducted studies based on all contact with health services, using standardised diagnostic criteria and free of numerator/denominator bias, also show similar findings (Bhugra *et al.* 1997; Commander *et al.* 1997; Cope 1989; Davies *et al.* 1996; King *et al.* 1994; Harrison *et al.* 1988; Harvey *et al.* 1990; Hutchinson *et al.* 1996; Littlewood 1992b; McGovern and Cope 1991; McGovern *et al.* 1994; Sugarman and Craufurd 1994; Takei *et al.* 1998; Wessely *et al.* 1991).

On balance the evidence suggests that there remains a genuine unexplained excess of schizophrenia in African-Caribbeans, particularly in young men.

International evidence

Does the excess schizophrenia in British African-Caribbeans reflect high rates in the sending populations? Data for the countries of origin are limited, and cross-country comparisons are confounded by diagnostic differences and variations in the provision, affordability and uptake of care, particularly secondary care. The incidence of schizophrenia in Trinidad (Bhugra *et al.* 1996) and Jamaica (Hickling and Rodgers-Johnson 1995) is within the range reported by WHO's transcultural schizophrenia research programme covering developed and developing countries (but not the Caribbean), which found international similarities in the incidence and symptoms of schizophrenia (Sartorius *et al.* 1986). The incidence is also lower than the rates reported for British African-Caribbeans. Hospital admission rates for schizophrenia are lower in Jamaica than among British African-Caribbeans (Hickling 1991), although half of all psychiatric admissions are for schizophrenia, higher than the 12–14 per cent for English-born and similar to the 40–50 per cent for Caribbean-born people in England, and there is a preponderance of young men (Burke 1974; Hickling and Rodgers-Johnson 1995; Sashidharan and Francis 1993). Explanations for the high rates of schizophrenia among British

African-Caribbeans are likely to be found here rather than in the countries of origin.

The evidence about African-Americans is similar to research findings for Britain, with higher rates of diagnosed schizophrenia, out-patient attendance and psychiatric hospital admission compared with whites (Adebimpe 1984; Flaskerud and Hu 1992a; Jones and Gray 1986; Lindsey and Paul 1989; Sue et al. 1991; Snowden and Cheung 1990). African-Americans are also more likely to be given strong medication (Flaskerud and Hu 1992b), have multiple admissions (Lindsey and Paul 1989) and poor outcome (Sue et al. 1991), and be over-represented in those involuntarily admitted (Lindsey and Paul 1989; Snowden and Cheung 1990). However, a survey of mental disorders in the general population found no black–white differences in schizophrenia prevalence after differences in age, sex, marital status and social class were taken into account (Adebimpe 1994). As in Britain, there is debate about misdiagnosis, stereotyping, and racial bias.

Pathways to care

Whereas only two studies show an absence of ethnic differences in routes to in-patient care, police involvement, and admissions under the Mental Health Act (King et al. 1994; Moodley and Perkins 1991), there is overwhelming evidence that, in comparison with white people, African-Caribbean people are:

- More likely to be admitted to psychiatric hospital following contact with the police and social services, less likely to be referred by their GP, and more likely to be detained by the police under the Mental Health Act (Bebbington et al. 1994; Bhui et al. 1998; Birchwood et al. 1992; Bowl and Barnes 1990; Commission for Racial Equality 1995a; Cope 1989; Davis et al. 1996; Harrison et al. 1989; McGovern and Cope 1987a; McGovern and Cope 1991; McGovern et al. 1994; McKensie et al. 1995; Moodley and Thornicroft 1988; Owens et al. 1991; Parkman et al. 1997; Perera, Owens and Johnstone 1991; Rogers and Faulkner 1987; Thomas et al. 1993; Turner, Ness and Imison 1992).

- More likely to be admitted compulsorily under the Mental Health Act as both offenders and non-offenders (Bebbington et al. 1994; Bhui et al. 1998; Bowl and Barnes 1990; Callan 1996; Chen et al. 1991; Commander et al. 1997; Cope 1989; Crowley and Simmons 1992; Department of Health and Home Office 1992a; Davies et al. 1996; Dunn and Fahy 1990; Ineichen, Harrison and Morgan 1984; Koffman et al. 1997; Littlewood 1986; Littlewood and Lipsedge 1981; Lloyd and Moodley 1992; McCreadie et al. 1997; McGovern and Cope 1987a, 1987b; 1991; McGovern et al. 1994; McKenzie et al. 1995; Moodley and Perkins 1991; Moodley and Thornicroft 1988; Noble and Rodger 1989; Parkman et al. 1997; Owens et al.

1991; Takei et al. 1998; Thomas et al. 1993, Turner, Ness and Imison 1992).

- More likely to be diagnosed as violent and to be detained in locked wards, secure units and special hospitals (Commander et al. 1997; Commission for Racial Equality 1995a; Cope 1989; Davies et al. 1996; Department of Health and Home Office 1992a; Dunn and Fahy 1990; Harrison et al. 1989; Koffman et al. 1997; Littlewood and Lipsedge 1988; Lloyd and Moodley 1992; McGovern et al. 1994; Moodley and Thornicroft 1988; Noble and Rodger 1989; Parkman et al. 1997).

Less well established is what causes these differences, whether it is greater prevalence of illness, more severe illness, delayed or inappropriate care, racism, or some combination of these factors. A comparative audit of acute admissions in two inner London districts concluded that the very high rates, particularly of formal admission, of Caribbeans were not explained by ethnicity (Bebbington et al. 1994). Research also shows that psychiatric diagnosis confirms the appropriateness of police referrals in a majority (about 90%) of cases (Dunn and Fahy 1990; Rogers and Faulkner 1987; Turner, Ness and Imison 1992).

Unfavourable pathways could be due to differences in the interaction with services at every stage of the illness (Bhui et al. 1998; Commander et al. 1997; Davies et al. 1996; Koffman et al. 1997; Parkman et al. 1997) – starting from low GP registration and under-utilisation of primary health care (Cole et al. 1995; Commander et al. 1997; Harrison et al. 1989; Health Education Authority 1994; Koffman et al. 1997; Odell et al. 1997), poor case recognition (Commander et al. 1997; Odell et al. 1997), and the interface between primary and secondary care (Commander et al. 1997). It is widely believed that community and primary health care services often fail to provide African-Caribbeans with the preventive and supportive care needed at an early stage to prevent the development of a crisis (Bhui et al. 1998; Bowl and Barnes 1990; Browne 1990; Cole et al. 1995; Commander et al. 1997; Commission for Racial Equality 1995a; Cope 1987b; Crowley and Simmons 1992; Koffman et al. 1997; Birchwood et al. 1992; McGovern and Cope 1987a; 1991; Davies et al. 1996; Department of Health and Home Office 1992a; Glover and Malcolm 1988; Harrison et al. 1989; Lloyd and Moodley 1992; Mercer 1984; Moodley and Thornicroft 1988; NHS Executive Mental Health Task Force 1994; Owens, Harrison and Boot 1991; Parkman et al. 1997; Perera et al. 1991; Rogers and Faulkner 1987; Sashidharan and Francis 1993; Thomas et al. 1993). When the crisis occurs, it is acute and all too often leads to intervention from the emergency services and compulsory admission. Adverse experience of psychiatric services and racism (Hutchinson and Gilvarry 1998; Parkman et al. 1997) may provoke alienation, poor compliance and loss of contact (Bhui et al. 1998; Davies et al. 1996; Parkman et al. 1997) – although some studies do not show a negative interaction with the service (Cole et al.

1995; Leavy *et al.* 1997). There is evidence that the key determinant of an adverse pathway (police involvement and compulsory admission) is not ethnicity but absence of family and/or social support and GP involvement (Cole *et al.* 1995; Davies *et al.* 1996). A high proportion (one-quarter) of African-Caribbeans live in single-person households (1991 Census), and African-Caribbeans with severe mental illness are more likely than other ethnic groups to be single, unemployed and living alone (Birchwood *et al.* 1992; Bhugra *et al.* 1997; Bowl and Barnes 1990; Glover 1991; Harrison *et al.* 1988, 1989; Harvey *et al.* 1990; King *et al.* 1994; Littlewood and Lipsedge 1988; McGovern *et al.* 1994, 1991; McGovern and Cope 1987a; Owens *et al.* 1991; Thomas *et al.* 1993; Wessely *et al.* 1991). Social isolation and the absence of a caring network may limit access to early and appropriate help, and increase the risk of statutory authority involvement and compulsory admission. Thus, a complex series of factors make the 'filters' between the community and hospital less effective for African-Caribbeans with mental health problems.

Just as African-Caribbean people are over-represented in mental health institutions, they are over-represented in the criminal justice process and the prison population (Bhui *et al.* 1998; Browne 1990; Department of Health and the Home Office 1992a; Wessely *et al.* 1994). Compared with whites, African-Caribbeans are:

- more likely to be subjected to stop and search
- more likely to be apprehended by the police on suspicion of committing a crime
- more likely to be remanded in custody and less likely to receive bail
- more likely to be assessed as mentally ill and subjected to compulsion
- more likely to be charged with a criminal offence rather than cautioned
- more likely to be given a custodial sentence.

Health and social services for mentally disordered offenders are discussed in a report produced jointly by the Department of Health and the Home Office (Department of Health and the Home Office 1992a), which expressed concern about the impact of custody on long-term outcomes and highlighted the importance of diversion from custody. This is particularly relevant since there is overwhelming evidence that African-Caribbean patients with schizophrenia have increased contact with penal and forensic services, and recent studies show their over-representation in prison (Bhui *et al.* 1998) and recidivist criminal behaviour (Wessely *et al.* 1994).

Case management

A common theme in the literature is that African-Caribbean patients are less likely to receive non-physical treatments such as psychotherapy, counselling and alternatives to institutionalised care, and more likely to receive physical treatments and strong medication (Bowl and Barnes 1990; Department of Health and the Home Office 1992a; Glover and Malcolm 1988; Littlewood and Lipsedge 1988; Littlewood and Cross 1980). Only one early study reported higher use of electroconvulsive therapy in African-Caribbean patients (Littlewood and Cross 1980), but there is some evidence that depot anti-psychotic medication is used more frequently (Chen *et al.* 1991; Glover and Malcolm 1988; Littlewood and Cross 1980; Lloyd and Moodley 1992). However, diagnostic differences explain some of this variation. Several studies show an absence of ethnic differences in treatment, or that where such differences arise they are explained by the more frequent diagnosis of psychosis (Dunn and Fahy 1990; McGovern and Cope 1991; McGovern *et al.* 1994; Perera *et al.* 1991; Chen *et al.* 1991; Lloyd and Moodley 1992).

Outcomes

There is growing evidence that African-Caribbean patients with schizophrenia have longer duration of hospital stays, higher rates of relapse/readmission, police contact, formal commitment and criminal conviction, and poorer social outcomes (Bhugra *et al.* 1997; Birchwood *et al.* 1992; Cope 1989; Crowley and Simmons 1992; Dunn and Fahy 1990; Harrison *et al.* 1989; Harvey *et al.* 1990; Lloyd and Moodley 1992; McGovern and Cope 1991; McGovern *et al.* 1994; Parkman *et al.* 1997; Thomas *et al.* 1993; Takei *et al.* 1998). Poorer long-term outcomes have also been reported (McGovern *et al.* 1994; Takei *et al.* 1998). A few report a milder course of illness and better clinical prognosis, although involuntary admissions and prison experience remain in excess (Callan 1996; McKenzie *et al.* 1995). Poorer outcomes could reflect ethnic differences in the nature and course of illness, interface with health services, inappropriate treatment, poor compliance, or lack of co-operation with a service perceived to be insensitive, coercive or racist.

In summary, African-Caribbeans have an excess diagnosis of psychotic illness and less voluntary contact with mental health services. Those with severe mental illness also have poorer outcomes, and are more likely than other ethnic groups to experience the 'revolving door' of cyclical transition between community, hospital and prison – clear evidence of unmet needs and deficiencies in care. Some of the ethnic differences in level and nature of illness, pathways to care, treatment and outcome can be explained by socio-economic factors, but unexplained variations remain. There is no evidence that differential misdiagnosis and management according to race explain the magnitude of the ethnic differences observed.

Suicide rates

Mortality statistics for England and Wales are available by the country of birth of the deceased, and not by ethnic origin. Analysis of suicide rates is, therefore, possible for first generation migrants, but not for UK-born African-Caribbeans. 1991 Census-based analyses for England and Wales show that suicide rates in Caribbean-born men and women in 1988–92 were lower than the national averages for males and females (Raleigh 1996) (Figure 3.7). 1981 Census-based analyses showed similar results (Raleigh and Balarajan 1992). Local studies confirm these findings (Neeleman, Mak and Wessely 1997) and also show low rates of attempted suicide among Caribbeans (Burke 1976a; McKenzie *et al.* 1995; Merrill and Owens 1987).

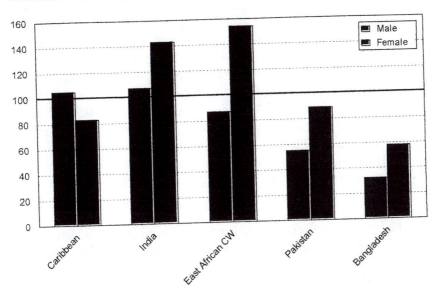

Figure 3.7

The suicide rates for West African born people are based on numbers of deaths that are too low for reliable comment. Most East African born migrants are of Indian subcontinent origin, and are discussed in the sections on Asians.

ASIAN PEOPLE

Prevalence of mental illness

The Asian community discussed here includes Indians, Pakistanis and Bangladeshis. It is important to remember that these groups, and the subgroups, are very heterogeneous in their socio-economic characteristics, lifestyles, cultural practices, health status and behaviour.

The evidence on mental illness in Asians is not consistent. Most research based on psychiatric hospital admissions, GP consultations, referrals to psychiatric clinics, and community surveys shows a low prevalence of mental illness in Asians, or rates similar to the general population (Cochrane 1977; Cochrane and Bal 1989; Cochrane and Stopes-Roe 1977, 1981; Gillam *et al.* 1989; Gowers *et al.* 1993; Ineichen 1990; Jawed 1991; Lloyd 1992; Stern, Cottrell and Holmes 1990; Thomas *et al.* 1993; Wilson and MacCarthy 1994). The PSI survey found low rates of psychiatric morbidity in Asians, particularly Bangladeshis, but noted doubts about the results because the mental health assessment instruments used were inappropriate for Asians (Nazroo 1997).

Other studies show higher rates of mental illness in Asians (Carpenter and Brockington 1980; Commander *et al.* 1997; Dean *et al.* 1981; Glover 1991; MacCarthy and Craissati 1989; Williams and Hunt 1997). The ONS survey noted an excess of depression among Asian/Oriental adults (Office for National Statistics 1995). Some studies show higher levels of stress in Asian women (Furnham and Shiekh 1993; Glover 1991; Glover and Malcolm 1988; Merrill and Owens 1986; Mumford, Whitehouse and Platts 1991; Perera *et al.* 1991; Williams and Hunt 1997), who are also at increased risk of self-harm and suicide (see section on 'Suicide rates'). Furthermore, it is frequently suggested that mental illness in Asians sometimes remains undiagnosed (see below). There is growing evidence also that alcohol-related morbidity is high in some communities of Asian men, particularly Sikhs (Bhui, Strathdee and Sufraz 1993; Cochrane 1977; Cochrane and Bal 1989; Dean *et al.* 1981; Mather and Marjot 1989).

Schizophrenia is diagnosed about 1.5 times more often in Asians than in Caucasians (Bhugra *et al.*; Cochrane 1977; Cochrane and Bal 1989; Carpenter and Brockington 1980; Dean, Downing and Shelley 1981; King *et al.* 1994; 1997; Koffman *et al.* 1997; Shaikh 1985); however, Cochrane and Bal have shown there is no significant difference when adjustments are made for age structure differences between Asians and whites (Cochrane and Bal 1987). King showed a significant excess of schizophrenia in Asians (King *et al.* 1994), although the findings for Indians and Pakistanis separately did not reach statistical significance and the seven Asians in the study included two 'other' Asians. On present evidence it is legitimate to conclude that schizophrenia rates in Asians are not significantly different from those in the white population.

Most research shows that compulsory admissions and police contact occur as often, or less often, among Asians as in whites (McGovern and Cope 1987b; Crowley and Simmons 1992; Bowl and Barnes 1990; Perera *et al.* 1991; Bhui *et al.* 1993; Shaikh 1985).

Explanations for low rates of mental illness

Various explanations have been advanced for the low rates of mental illness in Asians. They cannot be detailed here, but can be broadly summarised as follows:

- Genuinely low rates of mental illness, since the research reflects both community and other forms of care. The low risk is often attributed to the family and community support systems characteristic of Asian culture (Birchwood et al. 1992; Bowl and Barnes 1990; Cochrane and Stopes-Roe 1977, 1981; Gupta 1991; Ineichen 1990; Jawed 1991; Lin et al. 1991; Lloyd 1992; Nazroo 1997; Sartorius et al. 1986). Certainly, much lower proportions of Asians live in single-person households compared with other ethnic groups (1991 Census). The same explanation is often given for the favourable outcome and lower relapse rate in Asian patients with schizophrenia reported by many, including by WHO's transcultural schizophrenia research programme (Bhugra et al. 1997; Birchwood et al. 1992; Gupta 1991; Leff et al. 1990; Lin et al. 1991; Lin and Kleinman 1988; Sartorius et al. 1986; Verghese et al. 1989). However, many are sceptical of these stereotypes of Asians as 'psychologically robust'. For instance, Bangladeshis, one of Britain's most disadvantaged ethnic communities, are reported to experience higher levels of psychological distress than their indigenous neighbours, associated with chronic deprivation, language difficulties, poor and overcrowded housing, unemployment, social isolation and racism (MacCarthy and Craissati 1989).
- The reluctance of Asians to present with mental health problems (Beliappa 1991; Bhatt, Tomenson and Benjamin 1989; Bhui et al. 1993; Brewin 1980; Cochrane and Bal 1989; Gowers et al. 1993; Gupta 1992; Ineichen 1990; Jawed 1991; Krause 1989; Krause et al. 1990; Lloyd 1992; MacCarthy and Craissati 1989; NHS Executive Mental Health Task Force 1994; Sone 1992; Stern et al. 1990). This could happen because of any of the following reasons: psychosocial distress is not recognised or is perceived as physical illness, mental illness is stigmatised, illness is managed within the family, there is unawareness of local statutory services or they are perceived to be inappropriate, there are concerns about confidentiality, contact with male practitioners deters women, language and communication difficulties are a barrier.
- Failure of GPs to detect mental illness in Asians or to refer them to psychiatric services (Beliappa 1991; Bhatt et al. 1989; Bhui et al. 1993; Bowl and Barnes 1990; Brewin 1980; Commander et al. 1997; Furnham and Shiekh 1993; Gowers et al. 1993; Jawed 1991; Krause et al. 1990; Littlewood and Lipsedge 1989; Odell et al. 1997; Williams and Hunt 1997; Wilson and MacCarthy 1994). The

psychological expression of emotional problems is influenced by culturally derived concepts of illness and health (Bhugra 1997; Bhui and Bhugra 1997; Fernando 1988, 1991; Kareem and Littlewood 1992; Sashidharan and Francis 1993). In Asian cultures the well-being of the mind and body are seen as inseparable, and distress is not perceived as an illness. Psychosocial stress often manifests itself in physical symptoms (somatisation), as confirmed by numerous studies (Beliappa 1991; Bhatt *et al.* 1989; Bhui *et al.* 1993; Bowl and Barnes 1990; Brewin 1980; Cochrane and Bal 1989; Ineichen 1990; Jawed 1991; Krause 1989; Krause *et al.* 1990; Lloyd 1992; Mumford *et al.* 1991; Odell *et al.* 1997; Wilson and MacCarthy 1994). Language and communication difficulties could compound the articulation of such morbidity, as was evident in the PSI survey, even though interviewers and respondents were matched for ethnicity (Nazroo 1997).

International evidence

Research in India suggests that depressive disorders are as common there as elsewhere in the world (Sethi 1986). Surveys of mental ill-health in general practice in India report levels of 20–30 per cent, a significant proportion of which is undiagnosed (Sen and Williams 1987; Shamasunder *et al.* 1986); this is similar to levels in Britain (Brewin 1980). The incidence of schizophrenia in India, as reported by WHO's international study, is no different to other parts of the world (Sartorius *et al.* 1986). The balance of evidence suggests that Asians are probably just as vulnerable to mental illness as the general British population.

Suicide rates

Mortality statistics for England and Wales are available by the country of birth of the deceased, and not by ethnic origin. Analysis of suicide rates is, therefore, possible for first generation migrants, but not for UK-born Asians. 1991 Census-based analyses for England and Wales show that suicide rates in Asian- and East African-born men (most East Africans are of Asian origin) are lower than the national average for men (Raleigh 1996) (Figure 3.7). They are particularly low in Pakistani and Bangladeshi men, and are matched by low rates in the women. In contrast, Indian and East African women have rates significantly higher than the national average, detailed analyses showing that this excess is most marked in young women. Analyses for the 1970s and 1980s show similar patterns (Raleigh and Balarajan 1992; Raleigh, Bulusu and Balarajan 1990), notably high suicide rates in young Asian women, a consistent finding from national data covering three decades. The high suicide risk in young Asian women, including the UK-born, is confirmed by local studies (Neeleman *et al.* 1997), and is consistent with international literature (Raleigh

1996; Raleigh and Balarajan 1992; Raleigh *et al.* 1990). Burning is a commonly used method of suicide by Asian women (Prosser 1996; Raleigh 1996; Raleigh and Balarajan 1992; Raleigh *et al.* 1990).

Young Asian women also have higher rates of attempted suicide (Bhugra *et al.* 1999; Burke 1976b; Merrill and Owens 1986; Neeleman *et al.* 1996), although they are less likely to have a history of mental illness than white women attempting suicide. Social and family related factors are frequently cited as precipitators of self-harm in young Asian women.

CONCLUSION

Mental illness in black and ethnic minorities in Britain has probably been researched more than any other aspect of health in these communities. Yet, ironically, our understanding of it remains fragile and piecemeal. This is because, even in relatively homogeneous populations, mental illness is subject to greater complexities of causation, definition of what constitutes deviant behaviour, diagnosis and objective verification than most aspects of physical illness. These complexities are compounded when dealing with people of different cultures, in whom the perception and manifestation of mental illness may be different, and for whom English may not be the first language.

Earlier preoccupation with measuring the prevalence of mental illness in ethnic minorities has moved on to a concern about the ability of the NHS to respond to the differential mental health needs of diverse communities. This extensive review shows that mental health services often fail to meet the needs of ethnic minority clients. There is evidence of both over-exposure to acute services and the powers of compulsion, and simultaneously also of low utilisation, restricted access, poor case detection, and inadequate referral. The African-Caribbean experience of mental health services, in particular, remains one of the priority issues on the agenda of ethnic minority health in Britain. In no other aspect of healthcare are such profound ethnic differences apparent in the diagnosis, onset, course and outcome of an illness, and in the interface with services. The factors underlying this differential experience need to be investigated and addressed as a matter of urgency.

The challenge that lies ahead for the NHS is to provide mental health care that is responsive to ethnic difference. Fragmentation is neither desirable nor practical, given the diversity of ethnic groups in Britain, the marginalisation that would result for those that are few in number or geographically dispersed, and the implications for other health care provision. Instead, the goal should be to pursue the more difficult course of increasing awareness of and sensitivity to cultural differences within an integrated service that caters equitably to all members of our multicultural society.

ACKNOWLEDGEMENT

The author gratefully acknowledges the help of Helen Seaman and Kokila Chakraborty in compiling and presenting the material in this paper. This is a revised, updated and expanded edition of a summary report, *Mental Health in Black and Minority Ethnic People: The Fundamental Facts,* which was commissioned and published by the Mental Health Foundation in 1995.

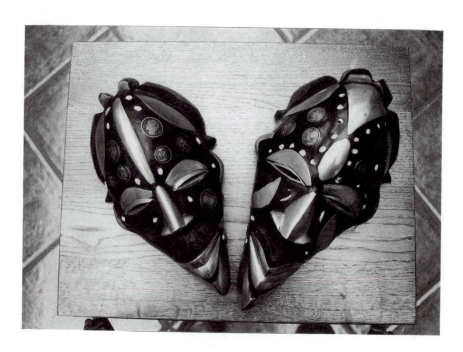

Two masks from Cameroon

CHAPTER 3

'Race', Criminality and Forensic Psychiatry

A Historical Perspective

Suman Fernando

INTRODUCTION

Psychiatry as we know it today arose about 300 years ago from two main sources: first, from the need to control and put away 'lunatics' who were disturbing, one way or the other, social order in European cities; and second, from a growing interest in matters to do with the 'mind' in European medical circles. As madness became a medical problem, 'illness' of the mind became the basic model for understanding people regarded by society as 'mad', and 'pathologies' (i.e. abnormalities) of different parts of the mind were postulated and elaborated – of emotion, of intellect, of beliefs, of feelings, of thinking, etc. Categories of illness were delineated and, gradually, a standardised classification system of diagnosis was developed. Some of these harked back to Greek ideas (e.g. depression, formerly called melancholia) but others (e.g. schizophrenia) were relatively newly formulated. Concepts of psychosis and neurosis developed and various theories about mind and illness of the mind emerged. But these disciplines did not develop in a social vacuum. Naturally the culture in which it developed played an important part in the ways of working and thinking that emerged – the culture of psychiatry. It is within this culture and reflecting this culture that the diagnostic system for the classification of 'mental illness' developed, that types of 'illness' were identified and judgements as to what is normal and 'pathological' were standardised.

We should note here that an illness model for human problems reflected in thinking, belief, emotions, etc. (i.e. one equivalent to psychiatry) did not develop in systems of medicine in Asia and Africa. Moreover, in these cultures the mind–body dichotomy does not dominate thinking about human life and its problems, and matters brought together (in Western culture) in psychiatry are seen in religious, spiritual, philosophical, psychological, ethical or medical terms; in other words, psychiatry, from a non-Western standpoint, may be seen as a mixture of all these brought together for social, cultural and historic reasons. In Asian and African traditions health is seen as a harmonious balance between various forces in the person and the social context. The Chinese way of thinking sees all illness as an imbalance of *yin* and *yang* (two complementary poles of life energy), to be corrected by attempts to re-establish 'balance' (Aakster 1986); the Indian tradition emphasises the harmony between the person and his/her group as indicative of health (Kakar 1984); and the concept of health in African culture is more social than biological (Lambo 1969). Thus in Asian and African cultures, human life is conceptualised as an indivisible 'whole' that includes not just the Western concepts of 'mind' and 'body' but also the spiritual dimension of human life. Further, understanding about the human condition does not (in Asian and African cultures) divide up naturally into the fields of study designated (in Western cultures) as 'psychology', 'religion' and 'philosophy'. However, it should be noted that cultures are not static systems but are ever-changing, especially as communication, migration and travel have become easier over the years. So today, the terms 'Western' and 'Eastern' no longer refer to geographical locations but to states of mind and attitudes towards the human condition.

Psychiatry and psychology which developed in Western Europe during the eighteenth and nineteenth centuries are largely 'ethnocentric' in that their ways of thinking and 'culture' reflect one cultural tradition or group of traditions generally termed Western culture. In particular, these disciplines have failed to draw from insights and knowledge in Asian and African cultures. Another related aspect of these disciplines that emerges, especially if one examines their practical implications, is their racism. And this is not surprising if one considers them historically. Both disciplines developed together at a time when the powerful myths of racism were being refined and integrated into European culture – the time when 'scientific racism' developed and social Darwinism placed different races at different levels on the ladder of evolution.

In the nineteenth century, psychiatrists in the USA argued for the retention of slavery, quoting statistics allegedly showing that mental illness was more often reported among freed slaves compared with those who were still in slavery (Thomas and Sillen 1972). And it was at that time that the now infamous mental illness *drapetomania* was constructed – an illness diagnosed among black slaves which (according to Cartwright 1851) 'manifests itself by an irrestrainable propensity to run away.' When John Langdon Down (1866) surveyed so-called 'idiots' and 'imbeciles' resident in institutions around London, he identified them as 'racial throwbacks' to Ethiopian, Malay and Mongolian racial types – mostly, he said, they were 'Mongols'. And over fifty years later when Carl Jung visited the United States and found it difficult to understand how white Americans could be so different culturally from their racial counterparts in Europe, he concluded that they were affected by 'racial infection' from living too close to black people. 'The inferior man exercises a tremendous pull upon civilized beings who are forced to live with him' (Jung 1930).

The racist tradition of psychiatry that considers black people as underdeveloped white people began in the nineteenth century and continues into the present. Well into the twentieth century the brains of black people were reported on as being smaller (and therefore inferior) when compared to those of whites (Bean 1906; Cobb 1942). A standard text on adolescence published in 1904 described Asians, Chinese, Africans and Indigenous Americans as being 'adolescent races' (Hall 1904). The ideology that equates intelligence with 'race' began with *The Measurement of Intelligence* by Terman (1916), was revived in the 1970s by Jensen (1969) and Hans Eysenck (1971) and continues today (e.g. Murray and Herrnstein 1994; Rushton 1990).

On visiting the far east, Kraepelin (1904) observed that guilt was not seen in Japanese people who became depressed; and he concluded that they were 'a psychically underdeveloped population' akin to 'immature European youth' (Kraepelin 1921). The apparent rarity of depression among Africans was attributed to their 'irresponsible' and 'unthinking' nature (Green 1914) or their 'absence of a sense of responsibility' (Carothers 1953). In the 1950s, Carothers' monograph for the WHO called *The African Mind in Health and Disease* (Carothers 1953) concluded that the 'African mind' resembled that of a 'leucotomized European'. In the 1970s Leff (1973) analysed observations across the world to hypothesise that people from Africa and Asia and Black Americans (the politically 'Black') were similar in having a 'less developed' ability to differentiate emotions when compared with Europeans and white Americans.

FORENSIC PSYCHIATRY

In the early nineteenth century, psychiatry began to impinge on the criminal justice system and the subspeciality of forensic psychiatry gradually appeared. As this happened, two concepts began to affect psychiatric and psychological thinking in Western Europe. First, the idea of 'degeneration' became accepted as a basis for understanding both criminality and insanity; and second, the notion that criminality itself was in-born and recognisable by physical appearance – the concept of the 'born criminal' – became popularised by the new science (*sic*) of criminology. According to Pick (1989) *dégénérescence* (proposed by Morel in the *Treatise* published in 1852 (cited by Gottesman 1991)) 'was the name for a process of pathological change from one condition to another in society and in the body ... Madness for Morel and many of his colleagues could not necessarily be seen or heard, but it lurked in the body, incubated by the parents and visited upon the children' (Pick 1989, pp.50–51). Degeneration was not primarily a theory of madness alone but one that linked crime, insanity and race (Pick 1989). Lombroso's 'science' of 'criminal anthropology' combining a doctrine of 'atavism' – reversion to primitive stages of evolution – with the theory of degeneration, conceptualised 'degenerates' as evolutionary throwbacks and identified physical features representing 'race' that revealed 'the true criminal in advance of any particular action.' (Pick 1989, p.128).

The background in which these ideas arose in Western Europe is significant. In the nineteenth century Europe was experiencing rapid economic 'progress': industrialisation had taken off as a result of wealth derived from slave labour of Africans and the seizure of land and genocide in the 'new world'; and then loot from India and other South Asian countries as well as the fortunes made in the 'China trade' (based on drug trafficking) was flooding into some parts of Europe. But Europe itself was experiencing increasing crime rates and an apparent rise in the number of lunatics. Progress (in Western Europe) appeared to be matched by a seeming inability to control criminality and lunacy. Meanwhile, the ideology that human beings were naturally divisible into 'races' based on physical appearance (especially skin colour) and that these races were on a hierarchy of development (racism) had become well established during slavery and accepted as 'scientific' facts as a result of 'social Darwinism'. The concept of degeneration linked to racist ideas found a fertile soil in which to grow as a plausible explanation for the rise of criminality and lunacy in the face of 'progress'.

Morel's concept of degeneration and Lombrosian atavism became of 'undisputed importance in clinical psychiatry' (Pick 1989, p.50) from the 1870s onwards, during the time that forensic psychiatry emerged. Undoubtedly, they played a large part in the thinking that led to three important developments in Western European thinking: first, construction of 'schizophrenia' as an illness (thereby explaining the rise of insanity); second, the popularisation of eugenics as a remedy for social problems arising from criminality and insanity; and third, the rise of the Nazi movement as the political framework for controlling (what were seen as) threats to white European civilisation. The mental hygiene movement within mainstream psychiatry aimed at cleansing society of unwanted elements and eugenic policies for the resolution of social problems gathered support. In 1918, Kraepelin set up the German Psychiatric Research Institute in Munich and the main thrust of its Genealogical Department was to establish a data bank of people seen as 'schizophrenic' (Weindling 1989, p.384). The end results were the sterilisation campaigns of the 1930s and finally the actual medical killing of people diagnosed by psychiatrists as 'schizophrenic'.

The development of forensic psychiatry in the nineteenth century meant that an increasing number of people in English prisons and asylums were designated as criminally insane. The institutional response to this was the opening of two purpose-built criminal wings at the Bethlem Hospital in 1816 (Forshaw and Rollin 1990). In 1860 an Act was passed for the better provision for custody and care of 'criminal lunatics' resulting in the building of Broadmoor Hospital in 1863, Rampton in 1910 and Moss Side in 1914 (Gostin 1986).

As it developed, forensic psychiatry functioned by examining the psychological and social meaning of whatever constituted 'criminal behaviour' (in a legal sense) rather than the intrinsic nature of the behaviour itself, increasingly focusing on issues about 'dangerousness' of individuals to 'society', irrespective of the nature of the society. In other words, psychiatry (and forensic psychiatry) did not take an ethical position on what constituted criminality – it merely accepted the definition proposed by the state. And this is still the position. According to Foucault (1988) the so-called 'abuse' of psychiatry in the Soviet Union in the 1960s, when political dissidence was diagnosed 'mental illness' (usually schizophrenia), was a logical extension of this intrusion of psychiatry into the legal system. Today, assumptions about criminality and dangerousness to society are often made on the basis of 'clinical judgements' which are wide open to permeation by all sorts of influences that are active in society at large – including racism.

CONCLUSIONS

The culture in which psychiatry developed over the past 300 years played an important part in the ways of working and thinking that emerged – psychiatry was ethnocentric to European culture. Since both psychology and psychiatry developed together at a time when the powerful myths of racism were being refined and integrated into European culture, racist thinking became an integral part of the system of psychiatry that Europe developed and then exported around the globe.

Psychiatric interest in crime may be seen as the arrival on the European scene of what is now known as 'forensic psychiatry'. From the beginning, this type of psychiatry was associated with control in alliance with whatever forces happened to be powerful in the society concerned. The overt and deliberate combination (within forensic psychiatry) of social control with the practice of a medical discipline resulted inevitably in the confusion of roles for people claiming to be forensic psychiatrists – the confusion of punishment with therapy, judgement about (moral) wrong-doing with (medical) diagnosis, and clinical care with custody. However, it should be noted here that, on all these counts, the boundaries between general psychiatry and forensic psychiatry are far from clear and remain unclear to this day.

As psychiatric interest in criminal behaviour increased, Morel's degeneration theory and Lombroso's criminal anthropology worked in together in the late nineteenth century, laying the basis for the ideology that criminality and insanity were natural states – inherited states with racial bases. In other words, both criminality and mental pathology came to be seen as throwbacks to earlier stages of evolution – to primitive cultures, to primitive people inevitably seen in racial terms.

The historical development of forensic psychiatry ensured that it focused on the danger posed to society by individuals considered to be 'mad' and the 'illness' that naturally became the epitome of madness was schizophrenia. Nineteenth-century ideas of race dominated by racist stereotypes of black people, encountered in Asian and African colonies and the American continent, inevitably fed into building up racist images of criminality and madness, dangerousness and aggressiveness, under-development and primitive cultures. All of these in the final count have become the substance of what goes for clinical judgement and diagnosis in forensic psychiatry – especially the diagnosis of schizophrenia.

CHAPTER 4

Differences in Ritual
and Culture

P.Q. Deeley

In this chapter I will discuss the relevance of understanding culture and ritual to the diagnosis and management of mental illness. In particular, I will argue that culture is an important source of variation in many aspects of individual functioning both in illness and in health. I will discuss different concepts of what 'culture' is and how it constrains mind and behaviour in order to point out the limitations of some concepts of culture as well as the relevance of more recent models.

CULTURE AS 'BELIEFS AND PRACTICES'

The definition of 'culture' has inspired considerable debate in anthropology and the social sciences. As long ago as 1963, Kroeber and Kluckhohn were able to assemble 150 definitions of the term. One of the most widespread conceptions of culture is that it is a socially transmitted set of beliefs and practices shared by a group of individuals (discussed in Good 1995, p.37f.).

The view that understanding a patient's culturally acquired beliefs is relevant to diagnosis and management is widely accepted in psychiatry. For example, a delusion is defined as 'a belief that is firmly held on inadequate grounds, is not affected by rational argument or evidence to the contrary, and is not a conventional belief such that the person might be expected to hold given his educational or cultural background' (Gelder, Gath and Mayou 1989, p.13).

When this perspective is applied to psychiatry, understanding a patient's enculturated (culturally acquired) beliefs is important for accurate diagnosis (to distinguish culturally appropriate beliefs from delusions or overvalued ideas), to help avoid offence and establish a rapport, and to promote 'insight' and compliance with treatment (although it should be noted that 'critical theorists' have argued against using anthropological understanding to support what they regard as the irredeemably coercive and oppressive institutions of medicine and psychiatry – see Good 1995, p.59f.).

In a co-operative view of the relationship between anthropology and psychiatry, the aim of studying culture is to identify and list the beliefs and practices of a particular group which relate to the body and mind in sickness and health, or which could be misconstrued as delusional by a culturally naïve psychiatrist. The aim is to educate health care providers about the culture of their client group to facilitate diagnosis and promote empathy and a therapeutic rapport. An example of this approach is the book *Transcultural Medicine* (Qureshi 1994), which contains a considerable amount of information about variations in diet, traditional medical practices, sexual and religious taboos, family planning, psychiatric problems, and other health related topics in the UK's major ethnic groups. While some of this information is accurate and provides some sense of the variations between ethnic groups, it also contains many alarming (and speculative) generalisations. There are statements such as, 'the ethnic Asian will have strong views against euthanasia, abortion, and family planning ... Where British patients will have views of rational morality, ethnic Asians will follow strict religious thinking' (p.86); or 'an Eastern person likes constant conversation and does not appreciate periods of silence which are culturally part of the English way of relaxation and this can also cause problems in a multi-cultural social gathering' (p.53). The book also contains tables characterising differences between ethnic groups; for example, one table specifies the degree of 'morbid jealousy' (*sic*) likely to be found in a husband according to their ethnic group if a male doctor examines his wife (p.108).

The notion that culture is nothing other than a shared set of beliefs and practices can be criticised for several reasons, although it should be noted that some studies which describe cultural systems as collections of 'beliefs and practices' are in fact broader in their scope – for example, *Worlds of Faith* (Bowker 1983). The informants describe how religious perspectives and practices influence their experiences and actions in the different contexts of their lives, so illustrating the complex relationships between shared belief and individual interpretation, experience and action.

One problem with thinking of patients as belonging to a particular 'culture' with a characteristic set of beliefs is that it implies a unanimity or homogeneity of belief in a particular racial, ethnic or national group which belies the considerable variation in beliefs and attitudes that exists within any definable group. Some beliefs may not be characteristic of a national culture, but be typical of a subculture within a nation state (tribe, religion, sect, class, etc.), or of the 'microculture' of a family or relationship. Such beliefs might be, for example, that modern medicines cause illness, telepathy and clairvoyance are genuine phenomena which can be learned, veganism can cure metastatic cancer, alien abduction occurs, or that people can be victimised by witchcraft (all of which I have encountered in clinical practice). A practical problem facing a psychiatrist is to decide whether a belief expressed by a client which is not obviously typical of their larger culture could nevertheless be typical of a smaller group. Alternatively, a client's view of the world might represent an idiosyncratic extreme within their own culture but be nevertheless coherently or appropriately related to it (see Littlewood and Lipsedge 1989, p.208).

A further problem is that thinking of clients as belonging to a particular 'culture' can create expectations which the client may find stereotyping or patronising. Individuals vary in the extent to which they subscribe to or appropriate elements of the 'culture' associated with their ethnic or religious background, and may resent being implicitly expected to conform to it (for example, dietary restrictions, dress codes, prohibitions on alcohol, drugs, premarital sex, or particular religious or supernatural beliefs such as belief in reincarnation or the reality of demonic possession). The complexity of individual cultural affiliations is greatly increased as first and subsequent generations of minority groups interact with the changing contexts and cultures of their adoptive countries, as they or their children become locally educated, work, watch TV, and so on. While a given group may strive to maintain traditional cultural boundaries and forms, even this may produce a conservatism which becomes dissonant with the culture of their ancestral society (see Bowker 1987 for the conditions under which religious fundamentalisms emerge).

More fundamentally, the very notion that culture can be viewed as nothing other than a set of beliefs and practices shared by a particular group has been criticised in anthropology. In this view, the emphasis on 'belief' underestimates the extent to which many aspects of individual functioning vary with culture. I will illustrate this broader conception of the relevance of anthropology to psychiatry by discussing the 'meaning-centred' approach in medical anthropology and approaches based on Bateson's notion of an 'ecology of mind'.

THE 'MEANING-CENTRED' APPROACH
IN MEDICAL ANTHROPOLOGY

In the book *Medicine, Rationality, and Experience* (Good 1995), the anthropologist Byron Good argues for an alternative conception of the nature of 'culture' and its relevance to understanding illness. Good criticises the notion of 'culture as belief' on the grounds that this implies a contrast between the 'beliefs' of patients about their illnesses and the *reality* of psychiatric illness or disorder itself, which is disclosed in the terms and models of psychopathology and their procedures of diagnosis (and investigation, where appropriate).

In this view, to think of 'culture' as a set of beliefs about an illness implies that the phenomena of psychiatric disorder may evoke interpretations which are culturally standardised for a particular group, but which do not effect or contribute to the underlying phenomena themselves (except where culturally acquired beliefs become elaborated into overvalued ideas, or delusions). This in turn implies that culture is superficial in its effects on psychology and neurobiology, and that accurate diagnosis and explanation of mental disorders rests firmly with progress in the latter two disciplines.

Good contrasts this viewpoint with an approach which he and other anthropologists have been developing in medical anthropology since the 1970s which he refers to as the 'meaning-centred' approach. In this view, 'illness' and 'disease' are not seen as phenomena which exist in nature independently of human interpretation, but rather as 'explanatory models': 'complex human phenomena are framed as "disease", and by this means become the objects of medical practices' (Good 1995, p.53). Instead of illness and disease being regarded as external to culture, the main interest in this approach is to explore the relation of biology and culture: 'biology, social practices and meaning interact in the organization of illness as social object and lived experience. Multiple interpretive frames and discourses are brought to bear on any illness event' (p.53). Studies have attempted to investigate 'how cultural interpretations interact with biology or psychophysiology and social relations to produce distinctive forms of illness' (p.53).

This approach entails, then, that illness does not only *evoke* interpretive activity in its sufferers and those around them, but that such activities *contribute* to the presentation and course of illness. The phrase 'interpretive activities' refers to the range of ways in which illness is interpreted in a culture. It is appropriate to think of this as an 'active' process because the interpretations are typically made in the context of special settings and activities – for example, history taking, physical examination, high-tech investigations, possession states of ritual healers, reading astrological charts, and so on. Furthermore, even the informal attempts at interpreting the significance of illness experienced by a sufferer and their close community reflect ongoing attempts at interpretation employing culturally acquired concepts.

Studies in this tradition have shown that cultural 'idioms of distress' organise illness experience and behaviour quite differently across societies – for example Nichter (1981) shows how South Kanarese Havik Brahmin women in India communicate intolerable psychosocial distress in a range of ways. Common complaints of leukorrhoea or menorrhagia, for example, may be strategically presented to Ayurvedic humoral physicians who seek the causes of the responsible humoral imbalances in strained family relationships.

Alternatively, cultures may provide 'final common ethnobehavioral pathways' – for example, Carr and Vitaliano (1985) analyse the Malaysian syndrome of *amok*, in which a sudden homicidal mass assault follows an intolerable insult and period of brooding. They view it as a locally standardised form of behaviour in which individuals with a variety of psychiatric diagnoses have been shown to engage (for example, depression, schizophrenia).

Good (1995, p.53f.) also claims that 'profound individual and cross-cultural differences in the course and prognosis of major chronic diseases have shown to be produced by cultural meanings, social response, and the social relations in which they are embedded' (for example Jenkins 1991; Waxler 1977).

This 'interactionist' model entails that many aspects of individual functioning are conditioned by the culture in which a person develops. These cultural constraints produce locally and individually specific forms of disorder when interacting with biological or psychophysiological predispositions present in many human populations. The constraints imposed on brain function by some predispositions or derangements may be sufficiently uniform for the associated syndromes to be clearly related in different cultures (in the case of schizophrenia or depression, for example); yet the local presentations of disorder still reflect the embeddedness of the individual within a network of culturally patterned relationships and interpretive practices. In this sense, it is not just exotic conditions such as *latah* which are 'culture-bound', but rather *all* illnesses, since the individual functioning which is disrupted in organic or psychopathology is culturally embedded, as are the interpretations and socially organised responses which this disruption evokes.

INTERPRETIVE PRACTICES AND THEIR ANALYSIS

Good describes different methods of analysing 'interpretive practices' and how they constrain mind and behaviour. One approach is to elicit 'illness narratives' from clients or those around them to study interpretive practices. An illness narrative is a story related by an individual or group of an episode of illness from their point of view. Rather than being subjected to closed or specific questioning to elicit symptoms, the narrator is encouraged to relate their story of illness in terms of what is regarded to be its start, what caused it, how it progressed, how it has or should be treated, and what implications it has for the narrator and those around them. It provides a way of analysing the cultural patterns through which illness is experienced, interpreted and acted upon.

For example, Good summarises research conducted in the 1980s on Turkish narratives about fainting. The subjects of the narratives had been independently assessed by neurologists to determine whether or not epilepsy was present, and if so what type it was. The findings suggest that epilepsy belongs to the larger cultural domain of fainting, with five types of narrative typically encountered which 'emplot' the illness in characteristic ways, giving order and local meanings to the events being experienced.

The commonest plot was of fainting beginning with a major emotional trauma associated with a frightening experience or deep personal loss, followed by a prolonged quest for a cure. A second plot type was of seizures beginning with a childhood fever or with an injury, often with a theme of maternal remorse for failing to protect their children. A third plot type told of seizures beginning with no apparent cause, and tended to be 'medicalised' in its focus on tests and physiology. A fourth plot type was of women who 'told stories of lifetimes of sadness and poverty, in which episodes of "fainting" were prominent'; the stories were voiced in a rhetoric of complaint, linked onset to life tragedies, and were not associated with extensive care-seeking. Most of these narratives were related by women diagnosed with non-epileptic seizures. Finally, in some narratives seizure onset was related as caused by the evil eye or by *jinn*, and included visits to religious healers or shrines (Good 1995, p.147f.).

Good comments that a given narrative may predominantly be of one plot type but exhibit features of others, and that multiple interpretations and a 'network of perspectives' may develop around an illness within a family. He argues that this maintains the openness of chronic illness to the possibility of final explanation and cure, and notes that narrators of stories about chronic or relapsing illness are still 'in the middle' of the story. The narratives help to evaluate the potential sources of seizures or fainting, draw into coherent relationship a number of life experiences, and anticipate the probable course of the illness and potential sources of efficacy (p.148). It should also be noted that it is common in all human cultures for different explanatory models and modes of treatment to be pursued simultaneously or at different times in relation to illness (particularly chronic illness) – this phenomenon is described as *medical pluralism.*

Another method of studying 'interpretive practices' is 'semantic network analysis', which to this point has been particularly used in the study of 'physical' symptoms such as 'heart distress' in an Iranian town, for example (Good 1995, p.54). The aim is 'map out the symbolic pathways associated with key medical terms, illness categories, symptoms, and medical practices', in order to describe the 'domains of meaning associated with core symbols and symptoms in a medical lexicon' (p.54). Good argues that this research shows that illness as a 'syndrome of meaning and experience' is constituted by culturally acquired networks of associative meaning which link it to fundamental cultural values of a civilisation, with new illnesses (such as AIDS) being linked to pre-existing semantic networks (for example, attitudes about homosexuals or particular racial groups) (p.55).

A similar approach is the study of the 'explanatory models' of clients, members of their social network, and healthcare workers about their complaints or problems. This approach is particularly associated with the anthropologist and psychiatrist Arthur Kleinman, and has been developed since the 1970s (Good 1995; Kleinman 1988a, 1988b). Some explanatory models are typical of a culture (for example, abnormal behaviour interpreted as due to spirit possession, witchcraft, humoral imbalance, breaking a taboo), whereas others may be more idiosyncratic.

Interpretive practices and experience

The 'interpretive practices' revealed through the study of semantic networks, explanatory models and illness narratives are culturally variable, and a major theme of the 'meaning-centred' approach in medical anthropology is that such practices contribute to the *experience* of illness, and – therefore – the symptoms elicited by physicians or psychiatrists. This does not imply that experience is simply a cultural construct, but rather that it arises in the interaction between a developing nervous system and a culturally patterned environment, which includes the symbol systems which allow interpretations to be acquired, expressed and modified.

The notion that 'interpretive practices' structure experience provides a basis for understanding both the crosscultural and historical similarities in psychotic illness, for example, and the local and individual particularities of expression. A 'delusion of control' arising from a misattribution of internally generated action to an external source will evoke attempts at interpretation which draw on culturally acquired cognitive schemata (of the kind represented in explanatory models, semantic networks and illness 'plots') which can form the basis for secondary elaboration into delusional systems (for a model of 'misattribution', see Friston and Frith 1995). While this approach is insufficient to account for *why* delusions of control should occur, it does contribute to understanding the form of their presentation and their connotations for the client and their close community.

Interpretive practices and ritual

Good's use of the phrase 'interpretive practices' implies that the interpretation of illness is not merely given in the experience of illness, but is an active, ongoing process for the sick person and those around them. Interpretive practices are similar to rituals, and in certain circumstances can be regarded as rituals, or are incorporated into them.

The category of 'ritual' has been re-examined in recent years (Bell 1993), but remains an important focus of study in anthropology. A ritual is a culturally standardised or stereotyped pattern of action and/or speech which stands in contrast to routine activity and evokes or is assigned a special purpose or significance amongst its participants – familiar examples in the UK are weddings, baptisms or funerals.

The highly structured nature of rituals led Freud to compare them to the stereotyped behaviours of patients with obsessive compulsive disorder, giving rise to the most common use of the term in psychiatry today (Freud 1907). The performance of ritual is one of the strategies employed by individuals and communities to maintain a sense of security and effective action in the face of psychosocial stressors (e.g. illness, death). In this sense culturally transmitted rituals resemble the individualised behaviours used by obsessive compulsives to keep anxiety at bay.

However, theories of ritual in anthropology emphasise many more aspects of what rituals are and what consequences they have for their performers and participants. Rituals communicate 'information' about a society's understanding of the social and physical world (Leach 1976, but see Gay 1978 and Sperber 1975 for qualification of this notion); they provide a means of relating to the 'occult' world of magic or religion as envisaged by a society (Fortes 1966); they express and inculcate core values and beliefs of a society (Geertz 1973) and facilitate psychosocial adaptation during periods of individual or communal crisis or change (see Turner 1983, Bell 1993 and Bowker 1997, p.819f., for further interpretations and debate about the nature of ritual).

Classic studies of ritual of relevance to medical anthropology would be Levi-Strauss' study of shamanic ritual to cure arrested labour amongst the Cuna Indians of Panama (Levi-Strauss 1972), or Victor Turner's study of the cult of Chihamba amongst the Ndembu of Zambia (Turner 1957). In the latter, for example, an ancestral spirit is thought to attack the living through a wide range of illnesses and misfortunes which centre on reproduction (for women) and hunting (for men). An initiation ritual is performed for a person identified as afflicted by Chihamba, in which the afflicted is initiated into the cult of Chihamba, becoming a 'novice' and then an 'adept' in that cult (Samuel 1990, p.87).

It is useful to distinguish between 'healing rituals', which are found in all societies in various forms and which are explicitly designed to heal illness, and other ritualised activities which may be performed to effect healing but may have other uses or significance as well – for example, fasting, prayer, or offerings (see Much and Mahapatra 1995 for an outstanding account of the practices of a *Kalasi* or possession oracle from Orissa, India). Kleinman has discussed the shared characteristics of 'symbolic healing' in different types of healing ritual or activity around the world, including secular activities such as psychotherapy. In Kleinman's view, healing depends on both parties to the transaction being committed to the shared symbolic order, whether it be sacred (e.g. exorcism) or secular (e.g. psychoanalysis). The skill of the healer consists in their abilities in word and deed to evoke optimism and belief in the efficacy of their practice. Key symbols are made relevant to the experience of the sufferer, and the sick person becomes convinced that transformation of their condition is both possible and happening (Kleinman 1988a, 1988b). Kleinman speaks of the 'psychobiology of hope and optimism', envisaging that the cognitive restructuring occurring through healing rituals may work in part through its autonomic and neuroendocrine effects.

This approach complements the theory called 'biogenetic structuralism', which has attempted to fashion a synthesis between anthropology and the brain sciences. In particular, the altered states of consciousness, cognition and affect often associated with the performance of ritual and crucial to its role in reinforcing or transforming psychosocial states have been a major focus of interest (D'Aquili, Laughlin and McManus, 1990; Turner 1983).

Understanding rituals performed in relation to the life crises experienced by users of health services (birth, illness, misfortune, death) is an integral part of understanding their 'life-world' (see Bowker 1983 for outstanding informant-based accounts of 'worlds of faith' in the UK). Ritual is also of potential interest to psychological medicine because of its efficacy in modulating the psychosocial and physiological state of ritual participants, as noted in particular by Victor Turner (Turner 1983) and the biogenetic structuralists. The ritualisation of behaviour is a highly conserved pattern in biocultural evolution, suggesting both that human beings are highly responsive to ritualised behaviour and that this responsiveness is incorporated into local adaptations to the social and physical environment. The loss or attenuation of traditional life-crisis rituals in some urban populations is one aspect of the breakdown of 'community' associated with urbanisation. The loss of traditional rituals, and the absence of ritual responses to novel stresses or life-crises of contemporary life (operations, 'empty nest', redundancy or retirement) may constitute vulnerability factors for psychological and physical morbidity (see Myerfhoff's work amongst the elderly of Los Angeles in *Number Our Days*, quoted in Turner 1980).

Understanding the mechanisms through which ritual affects biopsychosocial functioning may be relevant to developing new therapeutic interventions in medicine and psychiatry (a theme anticipated in Turner 1980). From this perspective, anthropological research is of vital importance to understand the efficacy (or otherwise) of the range of culturally organised responses to recurrent human problems as they are locally manifested.

It is also true, however, that formal ritual performances are not often encountered in the clinical setting of the ward, out-patients, or prison hospital (apart from religious services). The performance of ritual tends to be in the 'community', performed by users when they have returned there or by their relatives and close community on their behalf. The patterning of activity in hospital routines such as ward rounds or nurses' handover has led to the analysis of such occasions as 'ritual' (e.g. Goffman 1968). These occasions are clearly distinct, though, from the forms of symbolic action deliberately performed by clients and their community in relation to their problems as they perceive them.

It should be emphasised that cultural patterns are not only embodied in the more obvious and deliberate culturally organised activities such as ritual performances or open discussion of the causes of illness. They are also present in the subtle patterning of thoughts, feelings, conduct and relationships on a day-to-day basis. Shared patterns of symbol use and relationship are equally present, but are typically less obvious to participants and observers than more deliberate or 'special' rituals or attempts at interpreting or treating illness. This emphasises once again the importance of attending to 'interpretive practices' in the constitution of illness, but also leads to discussion of Bateson's notion of 'an ecology of mind'.

ILLNESS AND THE ECOLOGY OF MIND

Geoffrey Samuel has proposed a conceptual framework and terminology for modelling the relations between mind, body and culture based on Gregory Bateson's notion of an 'ecology of mind' (Bateson 1973; Samuel 1990). The 'ecology of mind' refers to this embeddedness of individual functioning within systems of patterned relationships and contexts. Aspects of individual functioning (such as cognition, perception, emotion, action) develop in culturally patterned environments and presuppose these contexts to 'make sense' and facilitate individual adaptation to the social and physical world. Samuel extended this framework of explanation by proposing a new terminology for modelling the relations between the characteristic modes of individual functioning and the contexts in which they are embedded (Samuel 1990).

For the present purpose, I will use the term 'conceptual framework' to describe a particular cultural patterning of thought, feeling, perception, action and relationships. In the same way that Good argues that 'interpretive practices' structure the experience of illness, Samuel argues that culturally acquired 'conceptual frameworks' structure different aspects of individual functioning. Thinking of individuals as possessing a repertoire of conceptual frameworks to enable them to function appropriately in the different contexts of their lives is consistent with viewing 'culture' as a heterogeneous phenomenon – a person can belong to different 'cultures' in different contexts and points in their lives. Furthermore, the range of cultures to which a person belongs (or the contexts in which they have learnt to function in culturally patterned ways) may not seem consistent or be predictable to an observer.

To provide a contrast to the difficulties of communication and relationship in a hospital or secure setting, I will discuss a type of relationship that was common in Kashmir until very recently. T.N. Madan studied the differing perceptions of Kashmiri society by its Muslim and Hindu inhabitants. The Hindu Brahmins formed a small minority in a society that was dominated by Muslims who did not accept or act on the basis of caste distinctions. The

Brahmins dealt with living in what the Muslims considered to be a non-caste society by treating the various Muslim subgroups they encountered *as though* they belonged to different castes, whereas from the Muslim perspective these groups were either occupational groups or did not in fact exist (see Samuel 1990, p.59f.). Samuel notes that 'the two groups managed to coexist in terms of two different social realities within a single society', and that 'the apparent conflict of conceptual frameworks ... did not lead to overt conflict' until Kashmir's involvement in the wider conflict between India and Pakistan (p.60).

Psychiatric wards and secure hospitals are also characterised by 'differing conceptual frameworks within a single social context' (Samuel 1990, p.59). What is unusual in the case of psychiatry is that the validity of the conceptual framework of the client is under scrutiny, such that coexistence despite difference is not an option if the difference is attributed to psychopathology (and particularly when the client poses a risk to self or others). Analysing clinical relationships in terms of carer and client operating within different conceptual frameworks in the 'same' situation provides a perspective on the special problems of this relationship. In fact, even members of the same culture can act on the basis of different conceptual frameworks in a given situation, but the problems of mutual understanding are compounded in cases where the framework of the other is especially unfamiliar.

One problem occurs where either carer or client 'frames' or contextualises the other's behaviour in a culturally inappropriate way. For example, I once assessed a Ghanaian woman who had been admitted under section several days previously with a suspected relapse of bipolar affective disorder. It was the first time we had met, and she protested that she was well and pleaded with me to let her go home. She knelt down before me and begged to be allowed to leave to return to her new job whilst weeping and praying to God, despite my embarrassment and attempts to dissuade her from this (she had recently found a job after months of unemployment). On reflection I interpreted her behaviour as an appropriate way of relating to authority figures in Ghana, in a situation in which a powerless woman's liberty is threatened (potentially for months, and possibly longer in her imagination), although I seriously considered the possibility that her behaviour was part of relapsing illness. She had certainly 'framed' her interaction with a British psychiatrist in an ineffective way, in so far as this behaviour would certainly be considered inappropriate in a culturally British person and could be considered evidence of emotional lability and disinhibition. In this example there was some uncertainty as to how to contextualise the other's behaviour, in my case because of cultural unfamiliarity and in her case either because of unfamiliarity, relapsing illness, or both.

In cases where diagnostic criteria are clearly fulfilled, this perspective can still provide a basis for understanding problems of mutual comprehension and enculturated differences in the 'same' situation. The psychotic patient can systematically interpret the 'same' ward environment in ways which reflect their delusional system and associated disturbances in perception, while the depressed patient can systematically interpret their environment in ways which confirm their depressive conceptual framework. This perspective can be linked to the approach of the 'meaning-centred' tradition described above, where illness interpretation and formation is structured by culturally distinctive semantic networks, explanatory models and illness narratives.

A more subtle problem is how the character and conduct of the client is assessed on the ward, where there is a shared conceptual framework of implicit moral judgement which is encoded in contrasts between 'mad' or 'bad', or in terms of whether a client's problems are due to 'illness' or are 'behavioural' (originally a morally neutral term derived from learning theory, but having acquired a sense of 'put on for particular purposes', often implying that the client's conduct is in some way deliberate and contemptible).

AWARENESS OF HUMAN VARIATION

One of the main problems for psychiatry of operating within the conceptual frameworks of a 'culture' is that they are inherently normative, often in subtle ways. This is true of any set of enculturated perspectives on the world, but in the case of psychiatry the cultural embeddedness of the practitioner may lead to systematic misjudgements about aspects of human variation which are typically devalued or pathologised in Western culture but not in other cultures (for example, trance states or visionary experiences – see Littlewood and Lipsedge 1989). I would argue that one of the principal roles of anthropology in psychiatry is to heighten awareness of the extent and depth of 'normal' cultural variation. The following examples have been chosen to illustrate counterintuitive normal variation under headings from the mental state exam.

Mood and emotion

Clifford Geertz described grief in a young Balinese man whose wife had suddenly and inexplicably died. He maintained a composed demeanour, greeting visitors to his house with a fixed smile and formally apologised for his wife's absence. He used locally learnt meditation techniques to try to 'flatten out … the hills and valleys of his emotion into an even, level plain' (Geertz 1985, p.128). Geertz contrasted this with his own (American) 'notions of the intrinsic honesty of deep feeling and the moral importance of personal sincerity' (p.128) to illustrate the depth of cultural difference between Balinese and American culture in the extreme situation of bereavement. It is interesting to note that as we in the UK become more 'American' (through media such as talk shows and soap operas, for example), traditional emotional responses to personal loss and sorrow which emphasise keeping a 'stiff upper lip' are less accepted and increasingly regarded as odd or even pathological. For example, the royal family was mocked and criticised in the tabloid press and in reported comments from members of the public for their 'unfeeling' formality and lack of overt emotional expression after Diana's death, particularly by travelling to their usual church service at Balmoral on the morning after she died and maintaining a formal demeanour.

Perception

In 'The illusion of reality or the reality of illusion', Al-Issa (1995) reviewed the evidence for the cultivation of visual and auditory hallucinations as part of culturally standardised modes of perception in different societies around the world. He argued that there is extensive evidence to suggest that hallucinosis is integrated into the normal range of experience of many members of non-Western societies through cognitive and perceptual training and does not imply pathology, although such cultural preconditioning may affect the presentation of psychopathology when it does occur (for example, in the content and form of hallucinations).

Cognition

The culturally acquired skill of reading affects cognitive performance on tasks of word and nonsense word repetition as compared to illiterate subjects who are otherwise culturally identical. Literate subjects perform better on tasks of nonsense word repetition, and it has been hypothesised that they are able to do this by virtue of an ability to process spoken words 'lexicographically' (i.e. how they are spelt) whereas illiterate subjects must rely on phonological processing alone. Functional imaging has demonstrated differences in the cerebral activation patterns of matched literate and illiterate Southern Portuguese women during performance of these tasks, which is one of the first studies demonstrating differences in neural organisation secondary to a form of cultural conditioning (Castro-Caldas et al. 1998).

Insight

In research conducted at the All India Institute of Medical Sciences in New Delhi (Deeley 1999) I elicited illness narratives and explanatory models from relatives of in-patients on the neurology and psychiatry wards. The interpretation of illness causation and the selection of appropriate treatment was frequently contested within families, where influential family members often make treatment decisions on behalf of the sick relative. A situation of 'medical pluralism' frequently existed, where multiple explanatory models and modes of treatment were adopted in succession or simultaneously. Medications were in some cases withheld from floridly psychotic patients for months because an influential family member attributed the derangements to spirit possession. 'Insight' – or concordance with the models of psychiatry – is affected not merely by the education and culture of patients but also that of their family and close community. Debate has arisen in medical anthropology and psychotherapy about the extent to which cultural differences in the interpretation of a client's predicament and problems should be taken into account in determining the goals of therapy and deciding what should count as 'insight'. For example, Littlewood refers to Hobson and Groves' work which uses 'the client's own explanatory models of distress to develop therapy in the individual context' (Littlewood 1992a, p.9).

CONCLUSION

In this chapter I have summarised and discussed concepts and evidence drawn from anthropology to explore the relationships between differences in culture and ritual and mental disorder. The view that culture consists of a set of beliefs and practices is too narrow to do justice to the extent to which individual functioning is affected by the interpretive practices and social relations of culture. Interpretive practices include the semantic networks, explanatory models and illness narratives studied in the 'meaning-centred' approach of medical anthropology. Bateson's notion of an 'ecology of mind' and its development by Samuel provides a theoretical approach to model the embeddedness of mind and body within the social and physical world. In particular, analysing the conceptual frameworks which structure individual functioning and relationships provides a basis for understanding the problems of mutual comprehension in a clinical setting. Finally, research on cultural variation serves to heighten awareness in psychiatry of the extent of normal human variation.

ACKNOWLEDGEMENTS

I should like to express my thanks to the following for their assistance and helpful comments: Charles Kaye, Dr George Stein, Professor Roland Littlewood, Professor John Bowker, Dr Maurice Lipsedge and Dr Nick Medford.

Thanks are also due to the Oxford University Press for their permission to use a quotation from the *Oxford Textbook of Psychiatry* (Gelder *et al.* 1989).

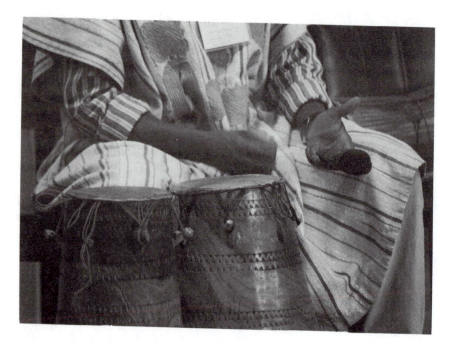

Musician playing on African Night, Broadmoor Hospital

CHAPTER 5

Racism and the Expression of Identity in Special Hospitals

Annie Bartlett

INTRODUCTION

In their book *Madness in America*, Gamwell and Tomes (1995) make several observations on the conceptualisation of ethnic minorities in the United States during the nineteenth century. They point out that amongst the psychiatric theories of the day was the idea that African-Americans freed from slavery were more likely to become mad and to require incarceration in hospital. Thus, the theory continued, slavery was good for African-Americans and kept them well. Second, they comment that where African-Americans were incarcerated in asylums that both 'northern and southern asylum doctors regarded racial segregation as a mark of superior management'. Third, they comment that the American specialists in insanity confidently described how American-Indians were unlikely to suffer from madness. Not only that, but this meant that the American-Indians could be moved off their historical lands because in contrast to European brains, American-Indians had small areas of 'concentrativeness', which meant they did not mind being uprooted, dislocated and deprived of their inheritance.

Such views informed the theory and practice of asylum psychiatry in nineteenth century America for many years. They are good illustrations of the retrospectively obvious connection between racist social attitudes and the practice of psychiatry. Such profoundly racist views are easy to spot today with hindsight. As we look backwards at historical practices it is easy to be complacent; current mental health practitioners can say in a self-satisfied manner to themselves that such things would not come to pass again. They would appeal to 'evidence based' practice and to increasing scientific rigour as if the naming of such totems were enough to protect professionals from the idiocies and unpleasantness of the past. In so doing, we forget that much of what we now so easily see as racist was described as scientific in the past, with such views being propagated by learned men.

I work for an organisation that describes itself as an equal opportunities employer. If I peruse the 'jobs for doctors' part of the British Medical Journal, almost all hospital trusts describe themselves along these lines. Perhaps a little conscious of their limited ability to deliver on the term 'equal opportunities', many suggest they are still working towards this desirable state. How far away they are is not so obvious to the hapless job seeker. In the last ten years I have sat on interview panels where the choice of interview candidates has never been made explicit and where the system of questioning was inconsistent. Data on the recruitment and retention of staff within any organisation in the NHS is, in my experience, available to very few employees. Historically the NHS has been poor at auditing the numbers of staff in its employ who come from any minority group and frankly dismal at examining the social processes that might go towards making a particular hospital a good or bad equal opportunities employer. Only since 1995 has collection of patient ethnicity data been mandatory in the NHS (Aspinall 1995; Hilton 1996).

Despite working as I do, as a white psychiatrist in a metropolitan, multicultural area, with large numbers of ethnic minority patients, cultural awareness has not been a mandatory element of my training. My capacity to deliver an appropriate service to individuals in my care which is sensitive to their cultural background is necessarily constrained by such gaps in my training. Though these are personal reflections, they are symptomatic of a general problem throughout the NHS. It may well be that there are many Trusts providing healthcare who are in essence paying lip service to the notion of equal opportunities. Concern about the experience of ethnic minority staff suggests that recognition and respect for cultural diversity is not necessarily being incorporated into training and practice in everyday work. This must be of concern in metropolitan areas where large proportions of the ethnic minority population live, but equally so in other areas where individual members of ethnic minorities will be more isolated.

In many ways therefore the well-publicised issue of racism in the special hospitals is not unique to the special hospitals. However, there are particular features of those units that make it yet more important that there is a vocabulary for the appropriate discussion of race, culture and ethnicity. This is essential to the provision of a culturally sensitive service to individuals which takes into account their cultural identity, however they see it.

This chapter will discuss first the nature and construction of cultural categories and their relevance to the practice of healthcare. Second, the relationship between the categories 'mentally disordered offender' and 'ethnic identity' will be briefly explored. Third, I will discuss how from the available literature we can see dilemmas for mental health care staff and patients in the special hospitals which relate to ethnic identity. Fourth, I will use examples from participant observation research in a secure hospital to describe the ways in which both racism and uncertainties about ethnic issues are apparent.

Starting with a theoretical approach, I hope to make sense of the empirical research that has been undertaken and to bring both understandings to bear on the practicalities of life inside special hospitals. Although people view special hospitals as, in some respects, hermetically sealed, it is axiomatic in this chapter that there is a crucial connection both for staff and patients between their experience of cultural diversity and racism outside of the special hospitals and what happens inside them.

WHAT ARE CULTURAL CATEGORIES AND WHY DO THEY MATTER?

This chapter is based on the idea that healthcare professionals have a duty to understand not only concepts of individual pathology but also concepts of society and culture, and cultural values. It is self-evidently unsatisfactory to identify patients as suffering from mental disorders such as schizophrenia because they have delusions and hallucinations but not be able to see other aspects of that person as important. It is helpful to take a holistic view and contextualise the person's illness in significant aspects of their life. This is a dialogue between patient and health worker. It takes the mental health practitioner into areas in which they may feel less qualified but which, if neglected, may do the patient a disservice. In general, mental health professionals receive disproportionately little training in social dimensions of mental health problems. A good starting place is a working definition of culture.

Any definition of culture is debatable (Clifford 1988). But culture can be seen as a combination, and indeed different combinations, of the things that people say, the things people do, the things people have and the things that people believe. The difficulty with such a simple working definition is that it can still be misused to produce cultural stereotypes that do not do justice to the complexity of a culture's or a person's identity. There are several safeguards against this. First, to remember that cultures differ from each other. Second, that cultures weight different aspects of culture differently. For example, one group of people may attach great importance to the land they live on, another will take pride in religious observance. The concept of cultural identity is helpful in encouraging all of us to think about what constitute our own cultural allegiances – is the football team more important than our work in determining our sense of self? Third, cultures change, and at different speeds, and in different ways. No culture is guaranteed to be stable or impervious to influences around it. Where people from different cultural groups find themselves together it throws up interesting questions of how to accommodate difference.

As Pfeffer (1998) recently pointed out, there have been significant changes in British public policy on race. After the Second World War, 'race neutrality' was favoured. This was followed by a recognition of minority disadvantage and support for assimilation of minority groups. The latest policy perspective is that:

> there is a recognition of the importance that people attach to having their distinctive identity acknowledged and respected, and moreover, recognition that the structure of British society and institutional racism both contribute to the disadvantages experienced by minorities.

Britain is a multicultural society. This is a confusing term. A quick glance back through British history will tell you that it always has been multicultural – Celts, Anglo-Saxons, Vikings, Normans, Catholics and Protestants all jostling with each other for the biggest coverage in the textbooks. Today multiculturalism means what in a sense it always meant, that we are a society characterised by a plurality of values, beliefs and behaviours. But currently, the cultural category we often invoke to divide ourselves into groups – because it means something to many of us – is ethnicity.

Belonging to a particular ethnic group, and we all do, will inform to some extent how we look at the world and ourselves in it. Components of ethnic identity will include shared language, a sense of place, religious or spiritual beliefs and cultural practices. The latter might include anything from food, to furniture, to how you will structure your family and other social relationships. As an individual you will choose which of these elements of this inheritance you want to retain – or you will feel it is not a matter of choice. In rejecting your origins you may still signal them. Other people may see you differently from the way you see yourself. To the Nazis, assimilated German Jews were not German but Jewish. Just as your own ethnicity will inform your sense of who you are, so too will it inform how you see others around you. For many white people in Britain, as for other ethnic majorities, seeing themselves as having an ethnic identity is curious. Indeed, arguably identity is more apparent when someone notices themselves as different from the rest.

But someone's total identity is a composite of a number of aspects of themselves, more or less apparent to them. For some people their work defines them in a way that is more important to them than ethnicity. For others social roles, e.g. being a father, can be what they value most about themselves. Thus the extent to which aspects of ethnic identity will encompass the whole of someone can and does vary.

The reason for dwelling on how culture and ethnicity in particular in this way is simple. Without a way of dissecting and discussing these issues it is hard both to share experiences and to see where we get things wrong. There are two ways of getting things wrong: either structural elements of the system of healthcare are discriminatory, or the intentional or deliberate actions of individuals are racist. Put another way, by virtue of occupying our own cultural niches, we all have ideas about ethnicity and they come to work with us. Because we are not necessarily aware of the values we hold, we may impose them on other people – particularly if we are powerful and they are not. Equally we may be aware of our values, believe them to be correct and impose them on other people who have perfectly good values of their own. The study of ethnicity is about the exploration of difference; racism is when that which is different is said to be negatively different for no good reason. The hard part is not so much recognising that obviously offensive terms about other ethnic groups are unacceptable, though those who defend these as humorous have some difficulty grasping this point. Rather, the challenge is to get to grips with the complex interweaving of social processes and attitudes, often unspoken and unacknowledged, that lead to social exclusion and alienation of certain ethnic groups.

MENTALLY DISORDERED OFFENDERS AND ETHNICITY

There is surprisingly little research into this area of psychiatry. In general, psychiatric research has examined patterns of presentation to services, e.g. hospital admissions, type of Mental Health Act section amongst psychiatric patients and apparent variation in the frequency of diagnostic category between ethnic groups (e.g. Harrison *et al.* 1988; King *et al.* 1994). There is less work on treatment (e.g. Chen, Harrison and Standen 1991; Noble and Rodgers 1989) and its relationship to the ethnic group of the patient, and a small amount on patient satisfaction (Leavey *et al.* 1997). Recently work on long-term prognosis and patterns of care has appeared (McKenzie *et al.* 1995; Takei *et al.* 1998). There is little work on the detail of the social attitudes and processes responsible for the apparently high prevalence of major mental illness in African-Caribbeans and disproportionate use of compulsory admission procedures (Cole *et al.* 1995). The stark conclusions of this research are well known, but beg more questions than the data can answer.

Specific research on 'mentally disordered offenders' and ethnicity has been scant but worrying (see Bartlett 1997). The pattern of overrepresentation of black ethnic minorities in compulsory care is continued and spans all levels of security in hospital. This echoes the situation in the criminal justice system which feeds the secure hospital system with requests for assessment and transfer (Hood 1992).

Increasingly, scepticism about traditional methods of inquiry has been voiced. The essence of this critique is that categories such as 'Afro-Caribbean', 'Asian' or 'White' are imprecise (Bhopal 1991; Bracken *et al.* 1998; Hutchinson and McKenzie 1995). It is suggested that the kinds of census categories used in much psychiatric research tell us little about how people see themselves and they fail to acknowledge that terms indicating an ethnic origin are socially constructed and mutable rather than biological givens. This last point is particularly important in health research as various branches of medicine, not just psychiatry, are interested in susceptibility to disease and its possible relationship to ethnic status. The validity of the categories is then vital to the quality of the research.

SECURE HOSPITALS AND THE CONSTRUCTION OF RACISM

For some time now the special hospitals have been heavily targeted for criticism. Report after report has criticised them, the impact of the reports spreading far and wide as scandal has been identified and disseminated by a story-hungry media. And yet they do not die. Both these observations are important. The 'Specials' are wounded animals, frequently assaulted but determined to carry on. One of the wounds has been to examine the extent to which any of the special hospitals permit, or even encourage, a racist culture.

It is intriguing to note that liberal commentators such as Gostin raised this as an area of concern over ten years ago (Gostin 1986, pp.70–71). He cites evidence from the inquest on Michael Martin, who died in Broadmoor, as follows:

> it appears that events leading to his death started with an argument between himself and another patient, who had been taunting him with racial abuse. Staff refused to intervene when asked to by Mr. Martin, who then took a swipe at a nurse, but missed.

What this excerpt highlights is that both staff and patients are capable of racism. But staff have an obligation, a duty of care to protect patients, including from each other. Patients do not have this obligation, and are sensibly construed as vulnerable. In this case staff omitted to act and this incident escalated, ending in the death of the patient. Interestingly, the bulk of the recommendations in the Ritchie report into Michael Martin's death are unrelated to the origin of this fatal incident and focus on the use of medicines and restraint techniques used by staff. This mindset is echoed in the 1988 HAS report on Broadmoor which neglects issues of racism entirely.

But by 1992 racism was firmly on the agenda. The Ashworth Inquiry stated in no uncertain terms, 'The culture at Ashworth nurtures covert and fosters overt racism' (Department of Health 1992, p.148). The evidence was that National Front literature was distributed with apparent impunity around the hospital and was seen by both staff and patients. A patient had received a death threat with an Ace of Spades playing card and a member of staff who had objected to the literature on display also received a death threat. Tellingly, neither the main hospital union, the POA, nor hospital management had taken any action. Concern about racist attitudes in staff was voiced in patients' letters to the Inquiry. The specific case of Handel Cascoe and his allegations of persistent racism by a member of staff illustrated the difficulties of checking facts in such a climate. If the allegations were true it also showed how ward atmosphere can be contaminated by small comments such as persistently referring to the black ball on the snooker table as 'the nigger'. It also indicates how in a restricted environment such as that of the special hospitals access to food of a kind you have been used to can be well nigh impossible. Other aspects of daily life can be made more difficult where staff are prejudiced against you.

The Special Hospitals Service Authority (SHSA) (1993) report into three deaths of African-Caribbean patients in Broadmoor picked up where Ashworth left off. At the time of the most recent death, that of Orville Blackwood, there was no Equal Opportunities policy in Broadmoor. The Inquiry team considered that 'Psychiatry is white, middle class and eurocentric', and that it was insensitive to the needs and views of ethnic minority patients in general and African-Caribbean patients in particular. It noted the 'filtration' of African-Caribbean patients into the secure hospital system, where people in positions of authority were unlikely to be from the ethnic minorities. In their view the organisational culture was characterised by the absence of an ethnic minority voice. Though not as scathing as the commentary on Ashworth, in seeing less evidence of overt racism, the criticisms were similar.

The essence of the two reports was that ethnic minority patients saw themselves as disadvantaged, and were, in a system not designed for them.

The policy response to these areas of concern is apparent in a variety of publications, e.g. the Reed Committee (Department of Health and Home Office 1992a), *Service Strategies for Secure Care* (SHSA 1995) and the Fallon Report (1998). Whether such policy is translated into practice is less clear at present.

In contrast to the regular inspection of each special hospital by the Mental Health Act Commission and the multiple published reports on their inadequacies, the plethora of medium secure units around the country, both NHS and private, have got off lightly. They seldom have to contend with the media spotlight in the same way. Recruitment of staff is likely to be local and this may be more congruent with patient populations than in the special hospitals. However, there is little room for complacency.

FIRST-HAND ACCOUNTS AND THEIR IMPORTANCE

Researching the areas of potential discrimination such as gender, ethnicity and sexual orientation is notoriously difficult. In a study in one of the special hospitals undertaken by the author and two colleagues in the mid-1990s no attempt was made to address the issue of ethnicity *per se*. Despite this, in the course of undertaking participant observation on three wards, the three researchers saw and heard information pertinent to this area. The reason for citing it here is because it enhances understanding of how ideas about ethnic minority staff and patients are expressed in the daily life of a special hospital. It also provides clues as to the way in which external concerns about this issue are perceived by staff in the special hospitals. In evaluating the significance of this material we encountered similar problems as faced by the Inquiry teams, i.e. incomplete information and difficulty in establishing how widespread were certain attitudes. The emphasis in this section is on how institutional racism can work; the data does not allow for sweeping generalisations about this special hospital or special hospitals in general.

Historical perspectives

Many male patients told us about their experiences of arriving at the hospital. They described their expectations at the time. Almost all patients were apprehensive about coming and some frightened, not least because of what they had been told about it. Common themes emerged from the descriptions of entering the hospital and their first weeks there. This was true despite very variable lengths of stay. A picture of an authoritarian ward emerged from these accounts; the indignities of this initial experience were evident to the researchers in the same way as they had been to the patients. At the same time the task for staff was rapidly to assess frightened and often mentally ill people coming reluctantly to an institution they feared. While that is true, the emphasis on 'them' and 'us' and the way in which the real imbalance of power appeared reinforced by this rite of passage must have particular meaning to individuals already feeling alienated from white society. The following man's account was particularly poignant in this regard:

> He told me of his arrival from prison 10 years ago. He said when he arrived that he was stripped naked and forced to get into a bath even though he had already had a bath that morning in prison. He said that he was called a nigger and that people were quite abusive to him. He said he was sure that it was not like that now, that was over ten years ago after all. But he said it was an enormous shock to him. His comment was that he was completely 'frit' by it. He said that his emotions were frozen at that point and his whole life changed in those first moments of his arrival. He said he lost the man who used to be and the man who could have been. The man who used to be may be waiting for him outside the gates but the man who could have been is gone, killed by Smithtown. He said he was glad to talk to me and he had not been so open about things for a very long time. He sounded quite surprised that he had talked like that to me and he said that I have not even asked him any questions and yet he still spoke to me. He said he wished he could talk to his RMO like that and explain the way he was feeling. (Fieldnote extract)

This was not a private conversation between researcher and patient. It was heard by a nurse whose comments at the end seemed to reinforce the patient's account as he said 'how terrible it was to hear stories about how things used to be' in the hospital.

Historical recruitment of black and other ethnic minority staff has been almost non-existent. One member of staff said she knew of two 'matrons' who said they would not employ black nurses and that racism used to be a terrible problem. She could see how black patients must have had a bad time. Several individual staff on different wards were identified by more than one informant for their racist views and behaviour.

What is hard to assess is the impact of these past episodes on the generality of the patient population and their sense of the present. Reports and inquiries tend to take a cross-sectional view, but individual people have long memories. The public nature of wards means incidents have large audiences at times. Indeed the historical prison literature suggests that inmates bring their past to bear on their prison existence; these experiences very much inform adaptation to a new secure setting (Irwin and Cressey 1962). This model suggests that many black patients would bring negative experiences of wider society and of the prison and healthcare system. They risk having had those experiences reinforced in the special hospital system; their memories of this will inform how they view the present regime.

Contemporary perspectives

There was one major public demonstration of unmistakeable overt racism in over 200 days of participant observation witnessed at first hand by the researchers. But there were aspects of the incident that pointed to a wider malaise. A member of staff told the following story:

> Mr Bloggs went to Majorca in spring for a golfing holiday and when he was there he was offered a robot to play with and he had an absolutely terrific game playing with this robot. So good that the following year he decided to go back to Majorca and again had a splendid game of golf with his robotic partner. He was so impressed by the quality of his playing when he was playing with the robot that he decided to go back again in the summer rather than the spring but when he got there and asked for his usual partner on the golf course he was told that they do not have robots in the summer because the sun is so bright it dazzles people. Mr Bloggs was a bit perturbed by this and said well why don't they paint them black and he was told that they had tried it but it was terrible, they had their hands in the till, robbing people, ripping them off (that is the punch line by the way). Around four white staff were there laughing appreciatively at this joke. (Fieldnote extract)

Not all the staff present laughed. But the story went unchallenged. It is interesting to pause, ponder your own reaction and contemplate what kind of work atmosphere allows this kind of material to be openly aired. There was no suggestion that those who enjoyed the joke thought it in any way inappropriate, or were alive to the sensitivities of anyone who might object. And the story went unchallenged. This illustrates the dilemmas for staff who find themselves witnesses to such incidents. When this example has been used as teaching material the responses to this situation have been varied and the answers informed by the ethnic identity of the staff and their position in the staff hierarchy.

The culture of professional groups, if it means anything, should mean that they behave towards people in ways that conform to professional standards. Within mental health the dominance of the medical model has meant that the individuality of patients has been less important than their disorder. Disorder is supposed to be treated in a largely preordained way. This has paved the way for the argument that in treating people in the same way, in accordance with the medical model, an acceptable level of practice is ensured. There is a parallel here with the now discarded public policy of 'race neutrality'. The 'neutrality' of this approach is reinforced by the blanket institutional rules and regulations of the special hospitals. These have arisen through a peculiar mix of history, convenience and ideas about safety. They substantially disregard the individual. Cultural needs which fall outside of mental disorder, or the institutional mindset, are unlikely to be identified and perhaps not met.

In practice institutional rules can be bent (Goffman 1961). So, when patients see the system as unfavourable, i.e. they do not get a room, other people seem to get more clothes or better work opportunities, it is hard for them to know whether this is the arbitrary madness of an imperfect system or the malevolence of a system not only insensitive but actively discriminatory. Where researchers are told that black patients are neglected by staff or that incidents between staff and patients are magnified out of proportion because the staff do not like black patients it is very hard to assess the validity of the observations. That some patients hold this to be generally true, but hard to say for fear of reprisals, is important. It will affect the way they experience their care. The deaths of the three black patients in a special hospital were well known. It was interesting to us that only black and ethnic minority patients mentioned a fear of dying in similar circumstances.

There was scope for black patients to socialise together, though this was viewed with evident suspicion by some staff. In contrast, there seemed little recognition that white patients socialised together and that this tended not to be thought of as 'a gang way of acting' by staff. Our observations suggested that small acts of cultural solidarity such as playing dominoes, a regular feature of ward life on at least one ward, allowed people to be more themselves and their use of language and demeanour would change. Dominoes were more likely if black and other ethnic minority staff were on the relevant evening shift. As no such staff were regularly employed on two out of three of the study wards there was little opportunity to make comparisons.

The situation for patients in an ethnic minority of one was different and perhaps more lonely, particularly if exacerbated by language problems. Certainly the obvious efforts the hospital was making to address ethnic issues were directed primarily at larger ethnic minorities. Social events were organised which both educated about cultural difference and, to a degree, encouraged its expression as the following excerpt indicates:

> When we arrived at the [social event] Joe is greeted enthusiastically by a Rastafarian patient from another ward. Derek is wearing a smart looking sports jacket. Derek's friend says loudly, 'Hey! You showing the cloth.' They chat for about five minutes in a language which means that I (white researcher) pick up only the odd phrase … Derek and his friend are joined by an Asian Moslem staff member who jokingly berates Derek's friend for being a failed Moslem. Derek's friend asks the staff member in what sense has he failed. The staff member says that he was a Moslem and now he had renounced his faith for Rastafarianism. Derek's friend said that it is all the fault of the Home Office. He explained that when he first came to Smithtown he gave his religion as Rastafarian but he was told that Rastafarianism is not recognised as a religion by the Home Office so he put Moslem as the nearest thing to it. The member of staff said that Derek's friend should have been strong. Derek's friend said that he was now Rastafarian so it is OK. This conversation was on a very friendly level and the Asian staff member was encouraging Derek's friend. I got a sense that all three shared a sense of being members of marginal religious groupings. (Fieldnote extract)

Attempts were being made to obtain and use the views of black patients. This involved both a meeting of black patients and reflections on how such groups of black patients have been seen as threatening in the past. One of the issues for the institution was its willingness or otherwise to agree what were really ethnic issues. The institution had a considerable capacity to disallow ethnic issues as such, and to rationalise them as problems for the individual, or as breaches of institutional rules – which it was argued applied to everyone.

CONCLUSION

To conclude, it seems that one of the challenges for the special hospitals is to agree a vocabulary about ethnic issues. To do so they need to allow issues to be raised and spoken of freely. Where there is disagreement this has to be frankly aired. Our experience suggested this was much more likely to happen where ethnic minority staff were present. It signalled to the patients that it was possible at least to begin to speak openly on a topic that could provoke defensive attitudes in both staff and the institution as a whole. We saw pockets in time and in place where, paradoxically in a special hospital, members of the ethnic minorities were free to be themselves but also evidence that at times it could be dangerous to try.

The recommendations made in successive reports are on the whole admirable and, if energetically implemented, would create a workforce educated and able to provide a culturally sensitive service to a multicultural group of patients. It will remain true, however, that the special hospitals are inappropriately situated to serve the populations allocated to them and recruitment of a multi-ethnic staff group would be particularly difficult in at least two out of three of them. Also, the whole basis of psychiatric theory is Eurocentric and the diagnostic detail and process, as well as its conceptual underpinnings, do not happily apply when used universally. To address this requires not only the world of the special hospitals to think hard about what it does but also the rest of psychiatry.

ACKNOWLEDGEMENTS

Research conducted by the author and cited in this chapter was generously supported by a Health Services Research Training Fellowship from the Wellcome Trust.

CHAPTER 6

Experiences in France and England

A Patient's Perspective

INTRODUCTION

Some years ago, I was admitted into an acute admission unit in the heart of France where the standard of treatment was very good. Unfortunately, I am unable to compare my experiences in France with the mental health care in Great Britain because I have only known maximum security treatment here. Clearly, the stigma associated with mental ill health is pervasive and afflicts patients everywhere whether they are of ethnic minority origin or not.

HISTORY

Care for the mentally ill in France has changed dramatically in the last 40 years. Up until the eighteenth century, mental illness was considered supernaturally or unnaturally caused, the work of evil spirits or human moral corruption. It was not until the mid-eighteenth century that there was any progress with the introduction of new pioneering reforms by the well known French physician Phillippe Pinel (1745–1826) at the Bicêtre Hospice, just outside Paris, where he initiated the humane approach to the care and treatment of the mentally ill to overcome often widespread cruel treatment.

Pinel called for the abolition of archaic physical restraints and the introduction of 'moral treatment'. These reforms eased the difficulties of the mentally ill as preconceptions about mental illness began to break down and the treatment of mental illness started to acquire more recognition.

In spite of these improvements, throughout the nineteenth century and up to the mid-twentieth, the majority of the mentally ill remained in jails where the use of physical force was still rife and recourse to straitjackets or padded cells prevailed. The mentally ill were prisoners with no basic legal rights and were detained ostensibly for their own protection. Reasons for admission to hospitals were social: people like single mothers, homeless, gypsies and the feeble-minded would find themselves incarcerated simply because they did not fit into society. These mental hospitals were self-contained and often self-sufficient. Most had their own homestead/farmhouses and workshops, providing revenue.

Up until the mid-1950s, mental hospitals in France were practically prisons. There was virtually no treatment on offer. Staff employed to 'look after' the inmates were more akin to prison officers than nurses. However, mental health care has changed a great deal in the intervening 40 years with the introduction of drugs along with a more liberal and humane approach. Methods of management and treatment strategies have now been introduced into the mental hospitals.

Psychiatric hospitals continued, however, to be concerned more with containment than delivering treatment of patients. It was the policy of short-term gain for long-term pain and therein lay the rub. Indeed, one must emphasise that the psychiatric system in France did not and could not exist to satisfy patients' needs. Instead, it was patients' behaviour that had to be modified to fit the needs of the system. The psychiatric system in France was always guided not by a philosophy of care but rather by political and social necessity. Unfortunately, this created more problems for society than it has solved.

ETHNIC MINORITIES IN FRANCE: WHAT ARE THE PROBLEMS?

There are now 118 psychiatric hospitals in France, 20 of them run by the private sector psychiatric services. These figures do not include private practices, out-patient clinics and mental-health centres. In 1993, 832,600 people were treated for their mental health of which 564,800 (68%) were out-patients and 267,800 (32%) were in full-time care amongst whom 19 per cent were of minority ethnic background origin.

The ethnic minority population in France is three or four times more likely to suffer from serious mental illness than the indigenous population. It was suggested that the cause is not genetic or biological but rather due to stress and the conditions under which these minorities live.

To have a sound understanding of current mental health issues amongst the ethnic minorities in France, one must emphasise the appalling conditions under which a large number of these minorities live. Poor housing, social exclusion, deprivation, intolerance and especially racism are fundamentally responsible for raising the incidence of mental illness amongst these populations. The pervasiveness of racism amongst the French is depressing. Non-European French, foreigners and other ethnic minorities have become an object of vilification for the 15 per cent of the French electorate who vote for Jean-Marie Le Pen and his racist party 'Front National'.

As for the majority of French people, they would approve of a 'multiracial' society so long as the proper spirit of patriotism is displayed by these ethnic minorities. In truth the malaise runs much deeper and begs the questions about the general attitude of the French towards their own ethnic minorities and their constant obsession with 'Frenchness' and French values. The French see 'integration' of these minorities as the only road to acquiring 'Frenchness'. However, unemployment and the ghettoisation of suburbs predominantly peopled by these ethnic minorities explain the difficulty they experience when they seek to become integrated into French society.

The modern-day multiracial French society has created the need for additional adjustments when dealing with mental illness. Racism in psychiatric institutions is seen as a cause for concern. Ethnic minority patients have been treated with contempt and total indifference. Moreover, these ethnic minorities have not been using their local statutory psychiatric services for cultural reasons such as language barrier, shame, embarrassment, the old myth of containing illness in the family. In addition, they have had little faith in the psychiatric system as misdiagnosing was rife. For example, a type of behaviour which could be perceived as normal in these minorities was very often translated into symptoms of mental illness by predominantly white French doctors. The nub of the problem has always been: whose context would be taken into consideration when diagnosing an ethnic minority patient? Furthermore, certain types of treatment or therapy, such as psychotherapy, were considered as suitable only for white patients and therefore medication was the only 'solution' for the ethnic minority patients.

REFORM AND CHANGE

The health authorities drew on their experience of what had gone before in the psychiatric institutions and found that there was ample scope for the exercise of initiative to tackle racism. It was a tailor-made opportunity to provide better services to patients from ethnic minorities in psychiatric hospitals. Their prime requirement was to maintain credibility by ensuring that a proactive approach was taken in dealing with racial issues. This approach was dependent upon an effective education and training programme, promoting cultural awareness and addressing the complex and diverse therapeutic interventions required by this group of patients, as well as provision of non-didactic cultural awareness material such as posters, leaflets, magazines, etc. In addition to this, course materials were designed to be flexible in terms of both where and when one studies.

The mental health professional practitioners realised that in addition to all the psychological and social problems that the ethnic minority patients had, they also suffered the handicap of racism and discrimination. Therefore these must be taken into account as a clinical matter. This was a new ethos of care in which the cultural and social determinants are explicitly taken into account when dealing with ethnic minority patients. The nurse is encouraged to provide key support by taking the lead role in a broader primary care. It was essentially based on forging a good relationship between the ethnic minority patient and the nurse, and thereby developing expertise and understanding of the needs of this group of patients. Suitable nursing and medical staff from all communities, regardless of race and religion, were recruited.

There has undoubtedly been an improvement in recent years in the care of ethnic minority patients in psychiatric hospitals. Although racism is still present, it is much less overt. There has been a progressive change in attitudes and behaviour in psychiatric hospitals. Recruitment is more rigorous and selective. Generally, staff are more tolerant and open-minded now than they were fifteen years ago. There are now more and more staff with substantial mental health work experience in a multiracial environment working in the psychiatric system.

There has clearly been a willingness by the authorities to embrace and promote change. There is now in France a more holistic approach to treatment of ethnic minority patients. Some French psychiatric hospitals have even gained a reputation for excellence in a number of areas, particularly in delivering a progressive and innovative philosophy of care to this group of patients within an attractive and non-oppressive environment.

The health authorities in France are sensitive to the needs of their diverse ethnic minorities. There are now more and more intercultural therapy units or groups in which the clinicians are able to communicate and interact with patients from diverse backgrounds and cultures. Non-organic treatments such as psychotherapy and milieu therapy are now available and offered to patients from ethnic minority backgrounds.

To draw on my own experiences of the psychiatric system in France, I must state that personally, as an ethnic minority patient, I have never encountered racism or any other form of active discrimination. This does not mean that racism does not exist in the French psychiatric institutions. Throughout the entire time I spent in the admission ward, I was given a lot of help and support. The unit where I was had an excellent standard of care. Upon my admission, I was given an information dossier specifying exactly who the particular 'key worker' was, and also listing the names of all other staff normally employed on the ward, detailing their functions. It was helpful, particularly since, as a newly arrived patient, I was not familiar with the personnel on the ward. I was shown around the unit. I was given a single room (in France most psychiatric hospital accommodation is in single rooms). As for my treatment plan, it was drawn up by the consultant who took into account the recommendations of all the clinicians involved in my assessment. My family was also involved. The treatment plan was discussed with me at the time it was first drawn up, and each time it was reviewed. My designated 'key worker', who was responsible for implementing my care plan, was in regular contact with my family to keep them informed of my progress.

ETHNIC MINORITY PATIENTS
AND CARE IN THE COMMUNITY

For a lot of mentally ill patients, especially those from ethnic minority backgrounds, daily life outside psychiatric institutions can be a daunting challenge. The mental health services have been shaped in recent years to meet the needs of the local ethnic minorities they serve. This development is also part of a long-term trend to limit over-regulated state intervention.

Patients are generally helped much more in France and better prepared for an eventual release into society; thus contact with the outside world is always encouraged.

A lot of patients are placed in foster families to restore the balance in their life. The family remains an imperturbably solid institution in France and the strong community links also help the reintegration of these patients and limit the possibility of relapse. These foster families must meet a number of criteria set by the local health authorities. The foster families would be operating under close medical guidance and would always be in contact with the hospital. Whenever a home is needed to take someone in then the foster families have to apply. They are paid 600 French Francs monthly (around £60) by the local authorities to provide board and lodging. Patients are given responsibilities and daily tasks to undertake and are encouraged to lead a normal and independent life.

In today's cost-conscious world, this option saves the health authorities a lot of money as it is far cheaper than conventional psychiatric hospitals. The treatment of mentally ill patients in a community setting turns out to be a model of real community care. This devolution of responsibilities is matched with accountability for performance and the quality of care the foster family offers to patients. Hence, the presence of a designated social worker 'Assistant Social', acting as a regulator, can represent the interests of these vulnerable and often powerless people.

WHAT ABOUT BROADMOOR HOSPITAL?

Broadmoor Hospital Authority has a very diverse population of patients. Twenty-two per cent of its patients are from an ethnic minority background. There is clearly a willingness by the Hospital Authority to embrace and promote change in order to provide better services to its ethnic minority patients and, most importantly, to challenge racial discrimination and support initiatives to tackle it.

The bigotry that I come across in my everyday experiences varies from the gross to the minor. For example, one particular member of staff who worked in South Africa during the apartheid era, and whose actions seem racially motivated, has been particularly difficult to me. He uses endless ways to taunt and provoke me, such as intimidation and invasion of my personal space which

I perceive as threatening. Moreover, he has always been careful to excuse his behaviour on grounds of safety and security.

Another member of staff told me that it was unfortunate that Hitler had not finished his job in dealing with minorities! Also, on another occasion, he told me to my face that the state was wasting money on me and that if it were down to him most of us would be hanged. On several occasions, I have been asked by the same member of staff: 'Are you still alive?' when passing him in the ward corridor (in reference to his perception that I am potentially suicidal).

These are the gross examples but I find it is the 'drip-drip' effect of petty insults or ignorant remarks which tend to have the greatest effect in demoralising me. For example, the way some staff talk 'through' me and pretend I am not there when I approach them to request some assistance. There are also other examples when staff make insulting remarks in response to a television feature of my culture, knowing that I am there watching too.

It has to be stressed that I and my fellow patients come across a lot of sensitivity, kindness and understanding. I could not write this chapter if I did not attempt to balance the bad with the good. However, the bad staff have such a significant and unhealthy influence, often out of all proportion to their numbers, that their input to our care is malignant. It undermines everyone's efforts.

In the last couple of years, we have seen a slow but steady change with regard to recruitment. A comprehensive in-house training programme is now given as part of the induction course to the new recruits. There has also been the introduction of NVQs and training programmes in cultural awareness (Working With Difference). Staff are gradually more aware of the problems encountered by patients from an ethnic minority background. To this end, the prime focus should be to work with staff with a substantial work experience in a multiracial setting.

The Hospital Authority, via the Patients Education Centre and the purpose-built Staff Training and Education Centre, is encouraging initiatives to show its commitment to, and understanding of, transcultural issues and the value of cultural diversity. This has not always happened in the past. Events such as 'Africa Week' and the '50th Anniversary of the Independence of the Indian Sub-Continent' have been staged in the hospital to promote cultural awareness.

That is not to say that the present system is efficient. The existing training programme does too little to prepare the newly arrived staff, with no first-hand experience of high security care, to deal with ethnic minority patients. Therefore, an in-depth understanding and knowledge of the ethnic minorities' needs within a maximum security setting should be at the forefront of any training programme. This will enable the delivery of better therapeutic intervention to this group of patients.

Much work is still to be done by the Hospital Authority to challenge misconceptions and reduce racism and discrimination at all levels. The Hospital's policies often fail to filter down to the 'shop floor'.

DEDICATION
In memory of my beloved uncle Dr K.A. who passed away in Paris on 30 June 1998.

M.A. (NH2)

PART II

Seeking a Better Balance

CHAPTER 7

Developing a Mental Health Service for Ethnic Minorities

Albert Persaud

The last fifty years have marked a significant black presence in Great Britain. The postwar migration from the Caribbean can be said symbolically to be represented by the famous sea voyage of the *Empire Windrush*. However, the black presence in Britain has a much longer history that is hardly known and rarely recognised or indeed acknowledged. Historians will remind us that black people were part of the Roman occupation of Britain and there were large black communities which were deported by Elizabeth I in the sixteenth century. In the 1950s and 1960s the influx of black and ethnic minority groups was mainly from the West Indies, India, Pakistan and Bangladesh, Hong Kong and China. In the late 1960s there was a flow from East African nations. More recently, members of other groups have joined the population in Britain as refugees or asylum seekers, for example Tamils, Kurds, Somalis, Iranians, Bosnians, Serbs, Kosovans and Albanians.

No matter where people came from, the ethnic minority communities of Britain have enriched the culture by introducing their cultural tradition, language, creativity, music, literature, art and style. However, in spite of this we still refer to people today in Britain as ethnic minorities – as groups of people who are significantly different and thus should be treated differently from the ethnic majority rather than creating a tolerance of a multicultural, multiracial society. Many ethnic minority communities still feel and experience a struggle for justice, and experience social, education and health disadvantages, and thus demand political changes that act against hostile racism that can be experienced at all levels in the society.

MAKING SENSE OF THE EVIDENCE

There is a growing body of research evidence on ethnic minorities' health. Many commentators have questioned the methodology of the research and more significantly the conclusions being derived from these processes. What has emerged are clear differences and disease patterns in different ethnic minority groups. These differences relate to a wide range of factors. Why there should be such differences has yet to be fully established.

Undoubtedly ethnicity and culture is not the only factor. Ethnic minority groups are frequently marginalised in many areas. In addition to healthcare, deprivation, overcrowding and poor housing often disproportionately affect these communities and there is a considerable body of evidence to suggest that social and economic factors are key determinants of health.

Although research into ethnic minority health is welcome, the evidence is that in a significant number of studies the research is based on hospital care with an over-reliance on the use of hospital or service utilisation data. The NHS reform, *Modern and Dependable* (Secretary of State for Health 1997), describes a health service which is led by the Primary Care Groups. This is the opportunity, supported by the evidence of increased use of primary care by ethnic minority groups, to pursue a national agenda of primary care evidence-based research.

The health experience of different ethnic minority groups differs from that of the major population. There are three major reasons for this. The first is that the prevalence of several common diseases is greater in some ethnic minority groups, for example coronary heart disease, hypertension, mental illness and diabetes. Second, certain groups have inherited diseases which are racially linked, for example sickle cell anaemia and thalassaemia. The third reason describes ethnic minority patients as not having equal access to health services because of communication and cultural disparities, which, amongst other factors, can affect individual knowledge and perception of their rights.

THE MENTAL HEALTH CONUNDRUM

There have been a number of studies on ethnic minority mental health. Unfortunately, these studies have by all accounts focused on certain diseases, for example schizophrenia in young African-Caribbean men, which has produced a counterproductive argument in that it has stereotyped and marginalised these groups of people into a form of time capsule which needs gradually unlocking. There are some studies on post-natal depression in ethnic minority women, but very little on eating disorders and children's mental health, and indeed on an increasingly elderly population. It is still unclear how many elderly people from the ethnic minority communities in Britain are participating in the new dementia drug trials.

The evidence provides a compelling argument for change; not only in the way mental health services are delivered, but also in the way we understand and accept the cultural and spiritual characteristics of the varying groups of ethnic minority communities.

There are many academics, clinicians and managers in the health service who will argue that the interpretation of some of these studies are biased in terms of their methodologies and diagnostic interpretations. However, what is clear is that ethnic minority communities experience different aspects of mental health services in a wide and varying way. Bhui and Carr (1997) synthesise the findings as:

- Excess diagnosis of schizophrenia in Britain's black population, ranging from 2 to 7 times the diagnosis for white groups. African-Caribbean people have up to 13 times the admission rates for schizophrenia and effective psychosis compared to white people. African-Caribbean people are more likely to be admitted into a psychiatric bed under a section of the Mental Health Act 1983.

- In addition, black people are more likely to receive chemical treatment, for example oral or depot medication. Other studies have shown that African-Caribbean patients with diagnosed schizophrenia are significantly more likely than white to have a non-standard pathway into care. In other words they are less likely to be referred by general practitioners and more often have police involvement (McGovern and Cope 1987a, b; Owens *et al.* 1991).

- Asian women have an alarmingly high rate of suicide. Suicide in women aged 20–49 born in the Indian subcontinent is 21 per cent higher than the general female population; there is a threefold difference in the 15–24 age group; 20 per cent of these deaths are by burning (Balarajan and Raleigh 1993b). In contrast, suicide ratios for Bangladeshi, Sri Lankan and Pakistani born women are significantly low, although raised in young Indian and East African men. Suicide rates for Caribbean-born people are low but are raised in the 25–34 age group (Raleigh 1996).

There are wide variations across Britain in how mental health services provide for various ethnic minority groups. Although there are some excellent examples that have developed from a bottom-up approach, sustained by strong executive support, the underlying force for change seems to be caught in a particular chicane of problems that has yet to be disentangled:

- There is little evidence in terms of effectiveness of outcomes for treatment of mental health of people from the black and ethnic minority communities. There is little evidence that the Primary Care level of the NHS has responded to the needs of ethnic minority communities.

- The mechanism for rapport between Health Authorities, Primary Care and the local ethnic minority organisations and groups is not sufficiently well developed to allow for active consultation. Some work at improving access to mental health care has been undertaken across the country; however, the ethnic minority communities have not been sufficiently involved in providing options on mental health care services.

- Within Health Authorities, Trusts and Primary Care it is recognised that mechanisms for consultation with the ethnic minority communities are required but there is insufficient knowledge about how to proceed effectively. The vast majority of research on understanding disease and patterns for improving channels of consultation and access to mental health care have been done in those areas of Britain with high proportions of people from the black and ethnic minority communities. However, there are very few studies that focused on regions where the ethnic minority communities are small.

- Whilst a good deal of research work has been undertaken with a genuine view to improving mental health service delivery for people from the ethnic minority communities, it is now generally agreed that this work has been at best too general and lacking significant and effective impetus to achieve long-term changes. At worst it has pathologised or made problematic these communities and failed to address the issue of institutionalised practice.

- A considerable amount of work has been undertaken, largely with the majority of white indigenous population, to work towards appropriate effective and efficient services. However, there is a growing recognition across the country that, in order to provide effective mental health services with the total multiracial and multicultural population, there is a need for the development and maintenance of improved links with the ethnic minority communities which builds upon previous initiatives.

- People from the ethnic minority communities are increasingly expressing the view that they are not willing to have their mental health needs defined for them or have them discussed in their absence. This therefore presents a challenge for local mental health services.

CREATING A MODEL FOR THE TWENTY-FIRST CENTURY

The 1990 and 1997 Health Service reforms in the United Kingdom put a major emphasis on the process of health need assessment to use financial resources more effectively and direct efforts towards proven intervention. This means that the assessment of the health and social needs of any population is an essential and integral part of delivering quality services and care. This by implication implies that needs assessment for the minority communities is essential to developing a quality mental health service. The momentum created by the present government's policy in addressing social exclusion, inequalities, poverty and racism includes the wider social concerns for housing, employment and fairness. However, ethnic minority communities tend to be socially secluded, because of the marginalisation and the stereotypical approach towards implementing effective policies. The NHS reforms have attempted to identify ethnic minorities' health needs, but have lacked any coherent strategy to address racial issues across healthcare.

Earlier in this chapter a description was given of the disease prevalence in certain ethnic minority communities and inherited disease factors. The issue of racism in the NHS and in the wider society has not been addressed, either at a policy or strategic level. It is not sufficient to imply that ethnic monitoring is the answer to addressing the needs of ethnic minority communities, as it is centred only on in-patient care. The impetus for reform is now overwhelming, to create a fair and just society for the twenty-first century.

The proposition, therefore, at a government level, can be considered within the following framework. There needs to be a comprehensive health strategy for Britain's ethnic minority communities:

- The immediate focus should be on the needs of an increasingly elderly population and on the maternal needs of women and children.
- There needs to be a strategy on how to involve and engage the ethnic minority community in the planning, development and monitoring of mental health services.
- Ethnic monitoring should be refocused on primary care as there is an abundance of identified needs in this wider care setting, instead of the present focus on hospital care.
- There is a need for a comprehensive set of evidence-based quality standards on prevention, treatment, care and rehabilitation on the various ethnic minority groups who have a mental health problem. This should be a pivotal part of the new NHS Health Improvement Programme and Primary Care Group development.
- Training of professionals to work in mental health needs to be more articulated and reflected in the state finals examinations. Questions relating to promotion, prevention, treatment, care and rehabilitation on mental health for the various ethnic minority communities should be part of the test.

This five-point framework can form the basis of an inclusive government strategy, based on best evidence, to inform best practice in creating a fairer and just society at a more local level of Health Authority Primary Care Groups.

Following from the national framework, the criteria for a comprehensive, ethnically sensitive mental health service should be:

- There must be a holistic approach towards mental health which includes the individual's own value on health, illness, spiritual belief and healing processes. Complementary therapy should be included as part of a range of services that provide choice and access. Planning and developing mental health services must include the views of service users and the wider community. One of the success criteria should include the development and monitoring of quality standards by the community.

- Specific developmental projects, for example 'No, There's No Problem Here' (Persaud et al. 1998), must be developed by the community and receive sufficient funding and support to create long-term benefits in a sustainable, controlled way.

- The needs assessment must include the cultural richness of each ethnic minority community with regard to their value system, their beliefs, traditions and racial significance.

- Care must be commissioned and delivered using the best available evidence, which will include education and training programmes aimed at addressing issues of racial harassment and prejudices in mental health care.

- Lifelong learning must include both those who provide care and those who receive care. Those who provide care must have a better awareness and understanding to apply the appropriate sensitivities to the various ethnic minority needs. Those who receive care should expect to receive an ongoing awareness of the pathway or journey they will experience during their problem, in order to develop better coping strategies for the future. There must be explicit expectations of excellence in the development of quality standards, which are adequately performed, managed and measured.

CONCLUSION

Very few ethnic/cultural events are solely celebrated or enjoyed by the ethnic minority communities. Fundamentally, as a culture, each group believes in sharing and learning from each other. The impediment could be the lack of resources and attitudes that will create the momentum for change. Changes need to be supported by imaginative and pioneering thinking, which the ethnic minority communities themselves want to lead.

There is a political momentum to create the necessary reforms to improve mental health, the social structure and environmental conditions in order to achieve a just and fair society in multicultural Britain. Conceptually, there is no major disagreement with this argument. However, the momentum for change needs to be driven by a desire to accept that Britain is a multicultural, multi-ethnic society in which the plural aspect of living creates a richness and diversity from which everyone can benefit. A health improvement programme for ethnic-minority mental health should be an aspiration of a society that wants to address injustice, racism and prejudice in its attempt to improve mental health.

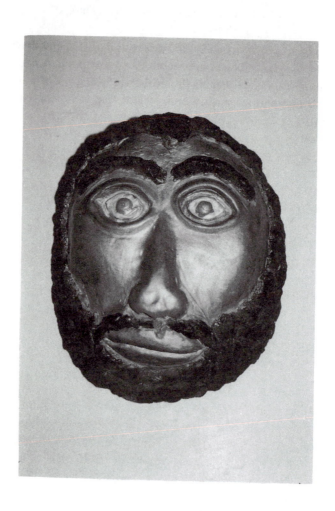

Bearded Face – David Usoro

CHAPTER 8

Supporting Black Patients in Secure Care

Legal Representation

Chinyere Inyama

INTRODUCTION: CHALLENGING DETENTION

Most patients admitted into hospital for psychiatric treatment are admitted there informally. The Mental Health Act 1983 (the Act) provides authority for compulsory detention via civil applications, criminal court orders, short-term powers and directions of the Home Secretary. Most patients detained in secure units are admitted by way of criminal court order or Home Secretary transfer direction.

Compulsory detention may be reviewed on application by a Mental Health Review Tribunal (MHRT) or the Hospital Managers (HM). Procedures adopted by the two bodies are similar but, in the context of detention in a secure setting, the MHRT is the most commonly used vehicle with which to challenge detention. The purpose of the MHRT is to safeguard against wrongful and unwarrantedly long detention and to generally protect liberty.

The application to the MHRT is made by the patient and, in some instances (e.g. Section 37 hospital order), by the patient's nearest relative. In cases where the patient does not apply there are provisions for automatic reference to the MHRT to ensure the case is considered at regular intervals by the Tribunal. Hospital Managers are responsible for automatic references of non-restricted patients and the Home Secretary is responsible for automatic reference of restricted patients. In addition, the Home Secretary may exercise his own personal freedom on the one hand bearing in mind the need for public protection allied with protection of the person from himself or herself on the other hand. The MHRT is expected to be able to make accurate predictions of the likelihood of repetition of the commission of serious offences and the understandable failure to do so in some cases has drawn criticisms. The criticism comes from a variety of sources and centres around a number of issues including concerns over a lack of nationally co-ordinated training programmes for the MHRT members, failure to adjourn after the patient's refusal to see a medical member and the need for the MHRT to have detailed information on the patient's index offence.

In a study commissioned by the Department of Health and Social Services and carried out by Jill Peay (1989) the main conclusions were that:

- Eighty-six per cent of MHRTs reached decisions that parallel the responsible medical officers' (RMO) view. Note, however, that there is massive regional variation.
- MHRTs often use retrospective strategies to justify their decisions.
- Common-sense attitudes are employed by MHRT members rather than them acting in strict accordance with the law.
- Caution was exercised in discharging dangerous patients. Note that race is often used as an index of dangerousness.
- There is often unacceptable delay in listing patients' cases for hearings.

The study also revealed different perceptions of the MHRT procedure by the participants, as follows:

- *RMO*

    - decried the adversarial attitude of legal representatives

    - felt the MHRTs damaged the therapeutic alliance between doctor and patient

    - felt there was undue diversion from their clinical duties

    - felt the MHRT were not accountable for the consequences of their decisions.

- *MHRT panel members*

    - felt they had insufficient training in mental health issues

    - felt they had limited powers except for making decisions to discharge or not to discharge

    - had no feedback on their decisions, therefore could not learn from mistakes.

- Patients

    - overall perception was that the MHRT was a fair and useful exercise

    - had low expectations of the outcome.

There is clearly a need to consider whether the time is now right for the establishment of an alternative procedure(s) to review detention, although the major priority of the present government is a root and branch review of the Act itself.

Law Society Mental Health Review Tribunal panel

Most patients now appearing before the MHRT are legally represented. Rule 10 of the MHRT Rules 1983 is concerned with representation and provides that patients who do not conduct their own cases can be represented by any person who they authorise for that purpose. Most representatives are solicitors, but they can include barristers, legal executives, and citizens advice bureau, law centre and hospital advocacy workers. There are advantages to authorising a qualified solicitor, not least the access to the legal aid fund (in order to instruct independent experts) and ease of access to MHRT documents not disclosed to the patient.

The Law Society administers a specialist MHRT panel of practitioners recognised as competent in dealing with MHRT work. The panel is non-exclusive and is open to solicitors, trainee solicitors, solicitors' clerks and Fellows and Members of the Institute of Legal Executives.

The scope of the panel is to provide expert representation to patients before the MHRT as laid down by the Act. A booklet listing panel members is circulated to the MHRT offices and Mental Health Act administrators of psychiatric units on an annual basis. To qualify for membership, the candidate must attend a full-day approved training course and have experience of representing a minimum number (4) of clients before the MHRT or have attended a similar number of MHRT hearings as an observer. The candidate must attend at least one Section 2, one Section 3 and one restricted patient hearing. The course content covers aspects of mental health law, medico-legal terminology, case studies, MHRT procedure, dealing with evidence and the role of the patient's representative. Once qualified, a candidate must then be assessed by way of application form, interview and, on occasions, references. The interviews are based on case studies and general questioning and successful candidates undertake to prepare cases and conduct MHRT hearings personally.

Membership lasts initially for three years and is renewable. Reselection is based on the number of hearings conducted during each three-year period. There are currently 360 practitioners on the Law Society MHRT panel list.

THE SOLICITOR'S ROLE

General points

The representative's role is to present a case for discharge (or otherwise) in accordance with the client's instructions. Rules governing the solicitor–client relationship are set out in the Law Society's guide to the professional conduct of solicitors. Generally, a solicitor is under a duty of confidentiality with his client but also owes a duty to act in the client's best interest as well as having an overriding duty to the court and judicial process. If, for instance, the solicitor is made aware that his client is exhibiting symptoms not detailed in the RMO report to the MHRT he cannot state that those symptoms do not exist since this would be positively misleading the MHRT. However, there are no easy answers and a solicitor must make a judgement on the weight he attaches to his various duties based on the circumstances of each case.

What is clear is that the solicitor is often the only person through whom the client expresses his/her wishes and views. As such, the solicitor must put forward his client's case vigorously and effectively. In order to do so the solicitor must gain his client's confidence by showing sensitivity to the client's situation and needs.

Legal aid

Initial preparation is generally carried out on the Green Form Advice and Assistance scheme. This is a means-tested legal aid scheme but will be free in most cases since most clients will be in receipt of qualifying welfare benefits. Preparation for and representation at the MHRT hearings is carried out under the Advice By Way Of Representation (ABWOR) scheme. This form of legal aid is non-means-tested and can extend to payments for independent experts. Solicitor firms exhibiting quality case, file and personnel management systems can apply for a legal aid board franchise, which is a badge of quality service. In the future, it is likely that only franchise firms will be able to carry out legal aid work.

Awareness of race issues

A joint Department of Health and Home Office discussion paper (1992b) stated:

- Black people are more likely than white people to be:
  - removed by police under section 136 of the Act
  - detained under sections 2, 3 and 4 of the Act
  - detained in locked wards
  - given higher doses of medication
  - diagnosed as suffering from schizophrenia or other forms of psychotic illness.
- Black people are also found to be less likely than white people to:
  - receive appropriate and acceptable diagnoses or treatment for possible mental illness at an early stage
  - receive treatment such as psychotherapy or counselling.

Further, a study by Cope and Ndegwa (1990) showed the following:

- Black patients are more likely than others to be admitted to psychiatric units from the prison system.
- Black people are significantly more likely to be diagnosed as schizophrenic and deemed to require transfers for urgent psychiatric treatment whilst on remand in custody.
- A larger number of black individuals receive restriction orders than their white counterparts.

A separate study by Browne (1990) showed that black individuals are more likely than white to be remanded in custody for psychiatric assessment by magistrates.

An earlier study by Cope (1989) showed that black people are more likely to be detained under the Act and to receive treatment in secure facilities.

There are conflicting explanatory models for black over-representation in secure hospitals. Fernando (1988, 1991) and Littlewood and Lipsedge (1982) attribute the over-representation to the inadequacy of diagnostic assessment methodology. Boast and Chesterman (1995) attribute over-representation not solely to misdiagnosis but also to the conditions of black people in British society.

Whatever the model, solicitors must be aware of these issues. Carefully taking instructions from the client and liaison with nearest relatives and other family members are vital in order to bring out race issues and set the context within which behaviour is exhibited.

Challenging diagnoses

The solicitor must be aware of the ethnocentricity of each of the recognised diagnostic classification systems and ensure he takes on board the fact that institutionalised racism can often impinge on the information collected by way of the client's history. The 1992 Ashworth Hospital inquiry found that, *inter alia*, there was evidence of extreme right-wing political activity and racist abuse by nursing staff (Blom-Cooper *et al.* 1992). The 1993 inquiry into the deaths of Michael Martin, Joseph Watts and Orville Blackwood at Broadmoor hospital found evidence of extensive institutionalised racism and that racist attitudes affected the diagnosis and assessment of black patients (Prins *et al.* 1993).

Accordingly, the client's comments on reports prepared for the MHRT should always be taken and inaccuracies and disputes noted and followed up. The solicitor must also be aware that the mental state examinations detailed in the reports will often contain a series of value judgements by the author incorporating stereotypes. Psychiatry can be accused of being used as an aspect of social control and a tool to medicalise morality, social and political issues. Knowledge and understanding of the cultural context of behaviour ensures the solicitor is better equipped to inform the MHRT of alternative interpretations of behaviour.

Challenging treatment

The Mental Health Act Commission *Third Biennial Report* (1989) and a study by Chen *et al.* (1991) concluded that blacks were more likely to be treated with drugs (and in higher doses) than their white counterparts. Solicitors should be aware of that fact and the stereotyping of the ability of black patients to benefit from non-drug therapy. Even when referrals are made to psychotherapy/ counselling services they are not usually culturally sensitive and are, therefore, of limited benefit to the client. Solicitors should make themselves aware of the location and organisation of culturally sensitive psychotherapy/counselling services.

Authority to incur the expenditure of independent psychiatry, psychology and social work experts on behalf of the client may be granted by the legal aid board. There are a slowly growing number of independent experts who are experienced in the transcultural aspects of the psychiatric experience and their reports can be presented to the MHRT as evidence. The legal aid authority can be further extended to cover attendance of the experts at the Tribunal itself so that the report's contents can be fully debated and taken into account by the MHRT in their deliberations.

CASE STUDIES

The practical aspects of representations of black clients incorporating the issues discussed can be illustrated clearly by the following case studies.

Patient X

This patient was born and brought up in South London with four brothers and two sisters as well as having a step-sister in Jamaica. His father had been absent from his home throughout his childhood. He left school at 16 without passing any exams and did various unskilled jobs. In the late 1970s he visited Jamaica for the first time, returning to England to train as a plasterer. He worked as a plasterer until he developed breathing difficulties and had to stop. Since then he did not hold down any regular job or perform any consistent work. He formed an interest in the Rastafarian movement and was sociable with girlfriends until shortly before his first admission to a psychiatric unit. He gradually withdrew into himself after several unpleasant experiences with police and the psychiatric services until a stage where he routinely kept himself to himself at home.

The client's view of his problems was that he had been getting migraine headaches for about ten years and getting stressed. He admitted to feeling low-spirited at times although he never had what could be described as clear-cut depression. When he withdrew himself from social life he then started taking drugs to counteract feelings of being miserable and fed up. He then got into trouble with the police over minor issues such as stealing milk or having small amounts of cannabis or speed in his possession. He remembered being sent to Queen Mary's Hospital, Roehampton, having being on remand in Brixton prison. Whilst in Brixton prison he felt he was roughly treated and had his dreadlocks forcibly ripped off his head. That experience left him very upset and probably resulted in his admission to hospital. Whilst in Queen Mary's he was injected with drugs which he believed added to his problems. He did not agree that he was mentally ill and felt that the medication which had been given to him did not help him. Two years before the Tribunal where he was represented, his younger brother died from suicide which upset and disturbed him greatly. Unfortunately, he did not talk to anyone about his feelings, including his social worker.

The discharge summary from Queen Mary's in 1990 noted symptoms of thought disorder and persistent paranoid delusions of being persecuted. No other symptoms of schizophrenia were noted.

The present admission had been initiated under Section 135 after a petition by tenants in the block of flats where he lived alleging that the client had been making noise for some months prior to admission. On admission, thought disorder, fluctuating behavioural disturbance and recent complaints from neighbours were noted as the reasons for his admission. He had been angry and hostile on admission but this attitude appeared to have settled over about a month after admission. The notes did not indicate any evidence of hallucinations or delusions but stated that he remained preoccupied with the injustice (as he perceived it) of the enforced admission. Also his thought disorder as evidenced by the use of neologisms was noted persistently throughout the admission notes. In the medical reports prepared for the MHRT the client's tendency to use made-up words, especially when he wished to emphasise something, was noted and attributed to thought disorder. The words he commonly used were 'razzle dazzled', 'abborted' (meaning abducted), 'ignorances', 'mental school-ups' (in talking about his education at school). He was in fact able to explain the meaning of the words in a sort of poetic fashion (i.e. related to sounds and bits of other words).

An independent psychiatrist experienced in transcultural issues was instructed. He noted the use of the made-up words and did not feel that the client's use of the made-up words/neologisms were indicative of a pathological process. The independent psychiatrist also stated clearly in his report that, from his experience, the diagnosis of schizophrenia was not justified in this case. He felt that it was given far too easily in the case of black youngsters and resulted in professionals not being sensitive to questions of depression and to psychological and social problems that lay behind the mental health problems experienced by people. He also felt that too great an emphasis was placed on medication that suppressed feelings and gave a false impression of improvement. The only symptom of schizophrenia consistently noted was the client's tendency to use neologisms, but the independent psychiatrist was advised by a psychotherapist who worked with people from a West Indian culture that this tendency to use made-up words was characteristic of conversation in some of the Islands and occurs in art forms such as rap and West Indian prose. In the independent psychiatrist's opinion, the client needed counselling in the first place although perhaps some medication (as a tranquilliser) may help from time to time. The main reason for the client's admission to hospital had been complaints from neighbours. This was clearly a social problem which could have been related to anxiety and perhaps depression resulting from his personal problems together with a bereavement reaction following his brother's death. The further conclusion was that the circumstances leading up to admission could have been better handled in a psychosocial framework rather than with compulsory admission and medication. The report was sent to the tribunal and the expert was called to present his evidence.

At the MHRT it was argued by the legal representative that the diagnosis was inaccurate and that this had been a case of the medicalisation of a social problem which should not have required compulsory detention.

The tribunal took on board the comments of the legal representative as well as the independent expert reports and decided to discharge.

Patient Y

This female client had a particularly difficult upbringing after having come to England from Jamaica with her siblings at the age of 5. Their mother had preceded the family out and established a home in England before the father came with their children. Both parents went out to work but the mother was the chief breadwinner. The father was aggressive to his wife and children. When the client was 9 years old her mother was killed in a fire at their home. Her death at the time was attributed to suicide but the client later learned, just prior to setting fire to her own flat, that her father was responsible for her mother's death. This information was relayed to her by the father himself and the fire-setting was a reaction to the confession.

An independent psychiatric expert was instructed and he noted that the summary of the client's mental health history indicated the appropriate overall diagnosis should have been recurrent depression or affective disorder and not schizophrenia. He noted that, as so often happens in the case of black people, the diagnosis of schizophrenia appeared to be given with very little justification, possibly because the client was unable to express her feelings very coherently whilst in a state of distress (misinterpreted as thought disorder) and had admitted to hearing voices on one occasion (a feeling which does arise in the case of severe affective illness). The independent expert further noted that the only symptom described on and off during the previous ten years had been thought disorder and there were no first rank symptoms of schizophrenia noted. In his opinion thought disorder is a very unreliable symptom on which to base a diagnosis since the judgement of whether it is present or not present is dependent on a close understanding of a language and a close rapport between the doctor making the diagnosis and the patient concerned. Also, in any case, confused accounts being given by someone in a state of distress can be very easily described as thought disorder quite inappropriately.

The MHRT absolutely discharged the client but made no comment about the possibility of misdiagnosis. The community mental health team treating the client carried on treating her as a schizophrenic patient. Unfortunately, the client committed suicide a few months after her absolute discharge. She had not received any specific treatment for her depression.

Patient Z
This male Nigerian client was admitted to a psychiatric unit in East London following relapse of schizophrenia. He had progressed well in hospital and was approaching a stage, according to his RMO, when he would be ready to be discharged. Her prevailing fear was one of the client absconding before the treatment plan was completed. This fear was based on the nursing notes and her own observation of the client applying lotion or cream on his body in preparation, it was thought, for an attempt to abscond. It was thought that the cream on his body would make him too slippery to be properly held by nursing staff, thereby increasing his chances of getting away from the unit. There was no comment in the nursing notes or the RMO report prepared for the MHRT about the fact that the client would dress normally after creaming himself.

At the Managers' Hearing, the representative introduced some personal evidence that he himself regularly applied lotion/cream to his body after bathing, since African-Caribbean skin due to its innate nature and the harshness of the water supply in many parts of England regularly needed rehydration after washing. The RMO was surprised at this observation despite professing to be a psychiatrist experienced in the treatment of black patients.

The client was discharged from his section by the Hospital Managers.

DISCHARGE AND AFTER-CARE

Progress through and eventual discharge from the psychiatric system depends largely on the co-operation with and take-up of after-care facilities. There is scope here for the involvement of solicitors in ensuring that the facilities on offer have a cultural relevance to the black client.

Any person admitted to hospital (whether their treatment is for physical or mental illness) may have a need for community care or health services in the community. In these cases, an obligation to conduct an assessment of those needs arises under section 47 of the National Health Service and Community Care Act 1990. In practice, the obligation to assess will be triggered in the cases of nearly all patients detained in special hospitals. The assessment must take place prior to discharge (in fact the assessment process should commence once a person has been admitted to hospital).

Policy guidance generally states that the decision to admit or to discharge from hospital is taken primarily on medical grounds but it also has to take into account social and other factors. Whenever these factors come into play, there should be close consultation between health authorities and social services departments. Subject to consumer choice, patients should not leave hospital until the supply of at least essential community services has been agreed with them, their carers and all the authorities concerned.

In addition, there has been much guidance issued in relation specifically to mental health patients and the requirement for a multidisciplinary assessment of need prior to discharge. This guidance includes circulars discussing the care programme approach, introduction of supervision registers, discharge of mentally disordered people and their continued care in the community and the *Building Bridges* document.

Unfortunately, the guidance is not often followed by health agencies and social services departments in making decisions regarding a person's future care needs and when decisions to discharge from hospital are made. The situation is further complicated since each agency involved has different and separate responsibilities for the provision of services and different budgets.

Solicitors representing black patients should ensure they are armed with information concerning culturally sensitive providers of community mental health and rehabilitation services. Solicitors should also be aware that anyone concerned with the welfare of a patient can request a care programme approach meeting. As the patient's advocate, the solicitor can request such a meeting and kickstart the multidisciplinary assessment and key worker allocation. He can also ensure that culturally relevant needs are kept to the fore in any discussion by attending each of these meetings. This work can be covered under the civil advice and assistance legal aid scheme.

The *Building Bridges* document contains the principles of the care programme approach and states that resources should be targeted on the severely mentally ill which will, of course, encompass many of those detained in secure hospitals. This is non-statutory guidance but can be enforceable by way of judicial review.

Statutory pre-discharge and after-care responsibility under section 117 of the Act can also be enforced through the courts. It should be routine practice for solicitors to ensure that a Section 117 meeting has taken place before the date of a MHRT so that the MHRT can make decisions after having as much information as possible laid before them regarding the possibility of treating the patient in a less restrictive setting.

Perhaps most importantly, the solicitor should always be aware that assessment of needs is only one issue. The most important issue thereafter is service provision. Solicitors should be familiar with policy guidance contained in the government publication *Community Care in the Next Decade and Beyond* (Department of Health 1990) where it was provided that: 'it is most undesirable that anyone should be admitted to or remain in hospital when their care could be more appropriately provided elsewhere' (para. 3.41) and 'Once means have been assessed, the services to be provided or arranged and the objectives of any interventions should be agreed in the form of a care plan. The objective of ensuring that service provision should, as far as possible, preserve or restore normal living implies the following order of preference' (para. 3.24). The order of preference is then given, beginning with support in the home and ending with the last order of preference as long-stay care in hospital.

It is clear that failure to make service provision decisions following completion of assessments too often consigns clients to long-stay care in hospital contrary to the above guidance.

CONCLUDING COMMENTS

Although law and psychiatry do not often make good bedfellows, it is incumbent on solicitors to act in the best interests of their client and according to the client's instructions.

It is clear that the key to effective legal support of black clients is in comprehensive training on awareness of cultural issues that arise throughout the whole hospital and community experience – from admission through to discharge back into the community. The training needs to be ongoing and regularly assessed for its effectiveness.

Solicitors generally need to be more proactive in pursuing patients' rights in hospital, in particular secure settings, where it is often presupposed by staff that patients' stays there will be very long term.

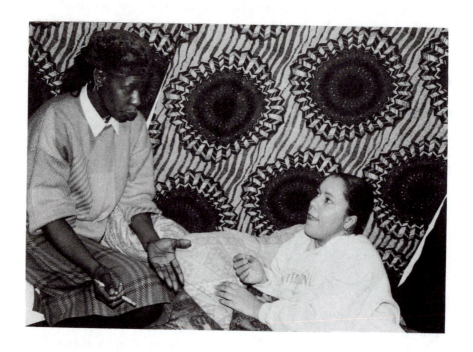

Conversation piece

CHAPTER 9

Change and Progress – the Right Pace?

Georgina Linton

This is no time to engage in the luxury of cooling off or to take the tranquillizing drug of gradualism. Now is the time to make real the promises of democracy.

Martin Luther King

PREAMBLE

I have been involved in one capacity or another with high security hospitals for more than fifteen years. In this chapter I will describe some of my experiences in relation to working with others to develop and implement an agenda which addresses the problems relating to the care and treatment of patients from ethnic minorities within these institutions. In identifying the major problems I perceive in this context, I aim also to describe the action that I consider needs to be pursued.

INTRODUCTION

The three high security hospitals, Ashworth, Broadmoor and Rampton have since their establishment held a particular intrigue for the general public, the media, politicians and healthcare professionals. The Mental Health Act 1983 defines the patients admitted to these hospitals as 'requiring treatment under conditions of special security on account of their dangerousness, violence or criminal propensities.' This description invariably conjures up images of people who are totally out of control, who pose a grave danger to themselves or the public and who are not particularly deserving of sympathy or empathy having committed heinous crimes. In many respects these images have contributed to the isolation and discrimination of patients receiving high secure care.

113

However, the fact is that there are a considerable number of patients currently in these hospitals who no longer require high security care. In addition, many patients have been placed in high secure care as a direct result of the failings of the general psychiatric services to provide the level and scope of clinical and therapeutic support required to ameliorate their mental health symptoms and enable them to continue living in a community-based setting. This of course may be partly due to resource limitations, as evidenced by the number of inquiry reports which have been published in recent years, highlighting the fact that a number of homicides committed by psychiatric patients could have been averted if an effective package of treatment and support had been provided much earlier.

The media has greatly influenced attitudes towards people with mental health problems and it has taken a particular interest in the high security hospitals. Whilst it is accepted that the media have a role and responsibility to report and comment on matters of public interest, the distorted and exaggerated reporting of mental health issues influences public perception of risk.

Nowhere is this more evident than if we consider the public/media response to black people who offend and are mentally ill. Against a background of heightened public awareness and anxiety about crime and the belief that the general public are at greater risk of violence by people with mental health problems, some sections of the media tend to emphasise the racial origin of individuals involved in acts of violence when these individuals are black. Black mental health service users are frequently characterised by racial stereotypes, i.e. being of considerable height and powerful build, requiring considerable precautions to be taken by professionals involved in their care. Such racial stereotyping should not serve any purpose in the clinical management of black patients in the community or within institutional care; however, the very powerful influence of the media impacts on even the behaviour of professionals. This is very likely to influence the decision-making process and contribute to black people remaining in institutional care for longer periods when compared with their white counterparts.

There is longstanding and increasing concern regarding issues relating to race and culture within statutory services and among black and ethnic minority mental health organisations. Research findings have highlighted the disproportionate number of patients from black and ethnic minority communities who are being treated in high and medium secure services. In medium secure services the current statistics are that black people, predominantly African-Caribbeans, are 30 per cent of the patient group, and in high secure psychiatric services this group numbers some 16 per cent. The high percentage of black males in high secure settings is frequently the focus of attention and debate. However, women within these settings are in a minority and thus the number of black women is even smaller, with the result that their isolation is even more acute. Recent research has found that many women who are admitted to secure psychiatric settings have experienced violence and abuse. Black women suffer the impact of discrimination both in terms of gender and race.

Despite these facts, the extent to which the various government policies and guidance are making a significant impact on the lives of these current service users in relation to their treatment, care and future service development remains patchy.

BACKGROUND

Although a registered psychiatric nurse in clinical practice for over 10 years, I had no previous contact or experience of working with people who were receiving in-patient high security care or had been through the system. However, I became increasingly interested in the care and treatment of ethnic minority patients admitted to the large psychiatric institutions, in acute settings and in the community. In the psychiatric service in which I worked, I observed that black and minority ethnic patients were often admitted to hospital in crisis, were prescribed higher doses of psychotropic drugs than other patients and discharged when still needing further psychiatric and social support which was frequently not provided. Many of the patients who were discharged relapsed while in the community, only to begin the same cycle again. The care and treatment of black patients appeared to be based on assumptions made as to what they are capable of and their ability and willingness to engage with services. In addition, the ever-present presumption of black people's propensity towards violence and aggression resulted in patients being moved on quickly, sometimes being transferred to locked wards or referred to medium and high security units.

With the encouragement of a particularly supportive and enlightened consultant psychiatrist I was encouraged to explore these issues further. The opportunity to work specifically on a change agenda which included influencing service development and delivery to black and ethnic minority patients arose when I was appointed as Development Officer to National MIND's (National Association for Mental Health) newly established three-year development project to focus on black and ethnic minority mental health issues.

The team, which comprised of three enthusiastic and committed individuals, began their work by extensively publicising the project's aims within both the voluntary sector network and the statutory sector. It was at this time that the team members began to receive correspondence from patients in the high security hospitals requesting visits, highlighting general concerns and on a number of occasions raising complaints. These three issues formed the basis of my initial contact and subsequent relationship with the high security hospitals.

WHAT I AIMED TO ACHIEVE

It is important to state here that I have had a variety of roles and responsibilities during my relationships with the high secure hospitals. My work on race and culture issues has been an integral part of my responsibilities. As I developed my interest in these issues so my level of knowledge and expertise increased. Increasingly, I and other colleagues were asked to offer support and on some occasions take a lead on these matters within the organisations in which we worked. The following objectives have been a consistent feature of the work that has been undertaken:

1.   Raise the profile of race and culture issues and establish the organisational agenda.

2.   Develop, in collaboration with key staff including managers, a service development strategy focusing on the needs of black and ethnic minority patients.

3.   Facilitate and support the implementation of strategies which would include services of direct benefit to patient groups.

4.   Establish contact with black service users so as to encourage participation in care planning and increase their contact with external support agencies.

EXPERIENCES

During the course of these early relationships a number of issues arose. These issues were mainly concerning the feelings expressed by black patients of isolation, low self-esteem and a belief that little or no attempt was made within the treatment regime to address, on an individual or group basis, their experience of racial discrimination, its impact on their mental health and their perception of the services offered to them. In reflecting these issues back to individual members of staff and clinical teams, the sensitivities of staff regarding this issue became apparent as concerns about issues of race and culture were perceived as a criticism of staff who are 'doing their best for a difficult group of patients'. There appeared to be a powerful notion that black patients had experienced discrimination through exposure to other agencies and that the services had no responsibility towards addressing these issues within the context of the patients' high secure care. The lack of knowledge about race and cultural issues within the services at that time, and in particular within clinical teams, was highlighted.

The development team decided to formalise their contact with the hospital by working closely with MIND's legal team who had established contacts and relationships with senior managers. This led to a meeting in 1995 between the then Chief Executive and the team where patient concerns were discussed and possible service responses explored. The need for a befriending scheme which included black and ethnic minorities drawn mainly from the London boroughs from which the majority of black patients originate, and the need for the development of a staff training programme addressing issues of race and mental health, were two of the ideas proposed.

It was acknowledged by the team that whilst these initiatives would be of benefit to the patients, other contentious issues such as seclusion and racial abuse were not being radically addressed. This was because the team were aware that access to the hospital to see patients and hold discussions with staff was not the automatic right of the voluntary sector and that relationships needed to be nurtured. Nonetheless, the team was able to make an impact by raising the concerns raised by patients, who had little confidence in the hospital's complaints process, with managers by working collaboratively with other agencies such as the Mental Health Act Commission. Issues regarding patients' rights, service delivery and complaints were raised with the Special Hospitals Services Authority, the Mental Health Act Commission and MIND's legal department. An outcome of this work was the provision of Afro hair and skin products within the hospital, improved access to religious and cultural leaders and the development of links with black and ethnic minority organisations. The team also provided support to patients through correspondence and occasional visits. This dialogue paved the way for further collaborative work. The subsequent death of two black patients in the high security hospitals led to independent inquiries which further highlighted issues facing black patients (and those campaigning for change) in the system, and allowed us to engage in initiatives which were clearly long overdue. The need to have a proactive approach to issues of race and culture in psychiatric practice was brought into sharp focus. The hospitals were prompted to explore frameworks of service delivery with external stakeholders as well as their own staff. Local MIND associations and black and ethnic minority mental health groups were encouraged to develop initiatives which would provide support to patients in high security settings.

The Secretary of State is keen to ensure greater representation of black and ethnic minorities as Mental Health Act Commissioners and my appointment to the MHAC in 1985 brought me into contact with a large number of black and ethnic minority patients. My role as a Commissioner enabled the commission to fulfil its remit in respect of meeting with detained patients, many of whom are black. In addition, in collaboration with other Commission colleagues, a Mental Health Act Commission Race and Culture policy was developed, a training programme instituted and race and culture issues were established as a feature of the Biennial Report submitted to Parliament.

EQUAL OPPORTUNITIES

The preferred approach to address issues of service equity, in terms of both human resources and service delivery, is the framework of equal opportunities. Equal Opportunity strategies have been developed by organisations to underpin policies and influence practice. However, progress on implementation of these strategies has been very slow and has met variable response from staff working in these organisations. People who have worked diligently within an organisation over a period of time, who believe that they have developed skills and expertise in their field, are unlikely to embrace the view that their attitudes, assessment, treatment and care in relation to the management of black patients is challenged. Thus when the issue of race, culture and mental health was raised within the context of the need for a greater understanding of the patient population in the high security hospitals, with the requisite service planning and delivery, a number of staff complained that their professional competence in providing care for these patients was being questioned. This in my view is because the majority of people consider themselves to be fair and committed to a policy of equality.

Latterly, I have experienced a readiness of staff to discuss these issues, to be involved in organisational and personal development programmes aimed at improving services. However, despite the various reports that have been written over the years which describe the effects of racism on the experience of black and ethnic minority people who work within the health service and who use its services as patients, there remains in some quarters a complacency regarding the action needed to address the issues. It appears that the participation in discussions about race and culture and the attendance at training events is treated as if it in itself represented the necessary change, rather than a prelude to such changes being introduced in the planning and delivery of services.

There have been considerable barriers to working to effect change within the hospitals. I would describe one barrier as personal/role conflict. This occurs often in the course of discussions with managers and staff concerning race and culture issues. I observe within the dynamics of the group that there is a general understanding of the issues but simultaneously a desire to detach the issues from organisational and individual practice. On occasion my perception of the discussion and response to the issues was that staff believe that I pursue the agenda solely through personal interest, and that the Race Relations Legislation and NHS guidance, as well as their organisational policies, do not exist. I have also experienced conflict when discussions expose a lack of personal commitment and awareness of race and culture issues. Some discussions became difficult when staff perceived that I was exposing their lack of commitment in bringing to their attention concerns raised by black patients.

A further issue is that organisations sometimes appeared to offload their responsibilities towards race and culture issues on to me as a black person. This creates a complex dynamic, as my interest and commitment stems in part from my being a member of the black community. On the other hand these fundamental issues which are underpinned by human rights principles of anti-discrimination, fairness and equity, were sometimes given a low priority and 'light touch' by white colleagues in organisations who seemed to be more concerned about the promotional value of their activity rather than fundamental change in organisational procedure, policy and practice.

The experience of black people in white organisations is highlighted by these dilemmas and conflicts. Although there are larger numbers of black professionals working in health and social service settings, few achieve positions of authority. Despite my various roles, including ones of significant influence, as a black person I am frequently expected to 'fit in' with the majority culture and not rock the boat, whilst at the same time I am asked to act as expert or advisor on race issues. This has been not only my personal experience but also that of colleagues (Fernando 1996; May 1994).

THE WAY FORWARD

The framework of law (Race Relations Act 1976) and government policy (NHS and Community Care Act 1990), as well as guidance issued by a variety of government or NHS sponsored committees (Reed Review; NHS Executive Mental Health Task Force 1994), focus on the need for services to be developed in consultation and partnership with black and ethnic minority communities to ensure that their particular needs are met.

Further work is needed to ensure that the rhetoric of collaboration, involvement and partnership becomes a reality both at strategic policy and planning level as well as local service development and delivery.

The responsibility for developing and implementing race and culture strategies should not rest only with black staff or those who are 'committed' to these issues. Chief Executives and managers should provide leadership by example, facilitating partnership arrangements across the black voluntary sector in liaison with key staff with an understanding of the issues. Managers and staff should be given objectives which reflect the organisation's aims, and the objectives should be monitored. The commissioners of mental health services should develop contract standards which translate the statements of policy into practice.

There is a need for the development of longer term medium secure settings and supported housing schemes which are able to provide the specialist support and treatment for people who often have a history of relapse of their mental illness. The core component of the service model within these facilities should be psychosocial. The model should address issues that are a frequent experience of black service users; these being loss, abuse, anger, family, unemployment, education, relationships and the wider concepts of illness. The longer term emerging mental health strategy aims to integrate the high security services with the wider NHS, thus ensuring that patients receiving high security care benefit from the full range of healthcare services as their clinical needs require them. In addition, the development of longer term secure mental health services for those whose needs are at present not met within high security facilities or by the limited length of stay in current medium secure services should result in a reduction in the number of patients in high security settings and the provision of more locally based services for patients who require a degree of secure care.

These proposals present both an opportunity and a threat. The development of longer term secure facilities may provide more opportunities for black patients to move more rapidly through the clinical pathway which integrates a rehabilitative process which is more community focused. On the other hand, it is possible that many more black people will be detained in secure psychiatric services in the future, because of a lack of well organised support services which involve health, social services, education and black organisations.

In my view there has been an over-emphasis on the development of facilities with insufficient details about appropriate service models for this group. The problem of the lack of appropriate community-based services to meet the needs of psychiatric patients is not particular to black patients. However, it is particularly acute for black patients who need to be transferred from medium and high settings. There is much that can be learned by the statutory services from the model of service provided by black and ethnic minority mental health groups in the voluntary sector. *A Consultation Event: The Future Provision of Secure Psychiatric Services for Black People* (Department of Health/NHS Executive High Secure Psychiatric Services Commissioning Board 1997), reported a more holistic approach to mental health. Listening, responding and working in partnership with black service users and their families is the key to effective joint working.

The mental health and well-being of black adolescents and the services available to them is currently a priority issue within the black community. There is concern about the increasing number of exclusions from school of African-Caribbeans, their contact with the criminal justice system and their consequent experience of mental health problems. Any strategy for adolescent mental health care must begin to address the root causes of the problems and experience of prejudice, superiority, disapproval and rejection faced by black youth in society today.

STAFF RECRUITMENT, RETENTION AND TRAINING
The high security hospitals are physically located in white, middle-class areas. Geographically they are some distance away from the inner city areas from which black patients are admitted. The majority of staff are recruited from the

local community with the result that the hospital workforce comprises staff to whom inner city life may be alien. There have been some attempts to increase the recruitment of black and ethnic minority staff to these establishments. Clarity about how the experience of these staff can influence the shape of the organisation, and provision of opportunities for training and development to ensure equality of opportunity in achieving promotion, is needed. The high security services should reflect the diversity of their patient population, as well as providing the opportunity for black and ethnic minority staff to contribute to clinical and therapeutic well-being of members of their community.

Black and ethnic minority staff need particular focus within the training and workforce planning agenda. During the recent celebrations of the 50th Anniversary of the NHS, I participated in a discussion with colleagues concerning the experience of black nurses who were recruited during the 1940s and 1950s to work within the NHS. It was felt that insufficient profile had been given to the contribution that these nursing staff had made to building the NHS. Often they worked within the least attractive disciplines within nursing, which at that time were mental health and learning disabilities, denied equality of opportunity in career development and promotion. A strong view was that the current shortage of nurses, and in particular mental health nurses, is in part a reflection of the poor experience of first and second generation black nurses who are reluctant to recommend the profession as a future career option for their sons and daughters.

There is a need for the UKCC to take a lead in developing guidelines for the development and delivery of a nurse training programme which includes focus on race and culture issues, its relevance to health and the setting of standards of competence for practice.

Race and culture training should be mandatory. The Mental Health Act Commission *Fourth Biennial Report* (1991) stated that 'many professionals lack basic knowledge about the different needs of ethnic minority communities and have little real understanding of institutional racism and the effect of cultural difference on the nature of mental disorder.' Research evidence should be utilised to develop training programmes. Staff should be able to demonstrate a clear set of competencies for working with patients which include awareness and sensitivity to these issues. The effectiveness of training and development initiatives should be monitored against organisational and departmental priorities. A key area would be change in practice and service delivered to patients through the Care Programme Approach, clinical supervision and the appraisal process.

There is also a need for more consistent organisational approach to the issues. There appears to be a perception of 'we've done enough, now we need to work on other priorities'. There is a danger that the activity itself rather than the achieving of defined outcomes will be seen as the end point.

CONCLUSION

I believe that it is quite possible to have innovation masquerading as change. My experience to date has been that mental health services have been excellent at espousing the rhetoric of equalities, participation and user involvement, without sufficient evidence of practice. Some of the achievements mentioned in this chapter started well only to flounder and then, with further prompting, begin again. In many ways this highlights the need for those concerned with anti-discrimination and anti-racist strategies to remain vigilant.

There has been some progress achieved in some areas in the treatment and care of black people in a high secure setting. However, progress has been painfully slow, and it would be not be an exaggeration to say that some patients have died for want of change. In the main the progress is the direct result of efforts made by champions for the cause of service equity. Two of the high security hospitals now have a strategy for the implementation of equal opportunities with a focus on both human resources and services development and delivery. These strategies have been ratified by the respective Chief Executives and have been translated into action plans. The impetus for this work, in my view, came from the High Security Psychiatric Services Commissioning Board's prioritisation of this issue, and collaborative work with the hospitals. The argument for integration of high secure services into the NHS has been well made. As we move towards the devolved responsibilities for commissioning of secure services it is essential that standards for service equity are retained within the overall contractual requirements, which are subject to the audit and monitoring process. The argument for an integrated approach will only be successful when organisations have achieved the level of maturity required to sustain the initial work done by those champions.

It is important to acknowledge the political, social and economic climate in which the changes that we must continue to make, take place. Brandon (1991) commented that, 'We are seeing the rapid psychiatricisation of ordinary human life, which conceals the overall deterioration in the quality of human relationships.' Thus in addressing the needs of people with mental health problems we need to work across organisational boundaries to tackle deep-rooted inequalities such as housing and employment with fair social policies which are the core component of a just and reasonable mental health policy.

PART III

Clinical Perspectives

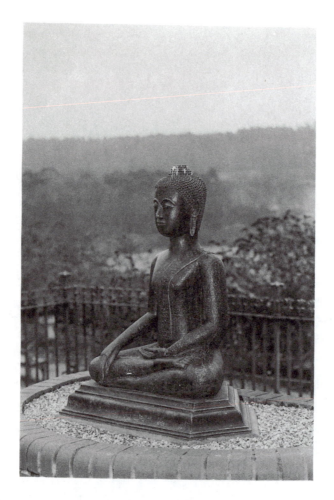

Statue of Buddha on the Terrace, Broadmoor Hospital

CHAPTER 10

Fair Treatment for Black Patients in Secure Care

Chandra Ghosh

INTRODUCTION

It has been my experience that psychiatry is and always has been a part of the establishment. The concept of abnormality of mind suggests a deviation from a recognised norm which is considered to be cross-cultural and acceptable by all societies.

I had the advantage of growing up in India and also of working in psychiatry there before I came to England in 1971. My first job was in Merseyside and the cushioned existence of a large psychiatric hospital did not in any way allow me to question my Eurocentric training. I had accepted the European concept of normative behaviour and nothing of my experiences in India had in any way questioned that acceptance.

Liverpool was a city which was very much like the city where I grew up, Calcutta. The Liverpudlians had the same capacity to cope with enormous stress and environmental deprivation through humour which was universal. The minority community in Liverpool, however, were conspicuous by their absence in Liverpool city. The joke about Upper Parliament Street, which was yellow at one end and black at the other, meant that there was an acceptance of getthoisation (of the Chinese community at one end and the African-Caribbean community at the other) that did not in any way question prejudice.

When I first started my Consultant job at a special hospital in Liverpool I was asked to look after men and increasingly had referrals of black men from London. The ward I worked on (in what is now Ashworth North) had a group of new nurse recruits who were mainly from Liverpool and who were remarkable in how non-prejudiced and non-judgemental they were in the way they dealt with the patients. It was only in the latter part of my ten years as a Consultant at Ashworth North that I began to question some of the attitudes and prejudices that my patients had been exposed to when they were living in the community, particularly in parts of London.

RACIAL PREJUDICE

I moved to Broadmoor Hospital in 1988 and initially was responsible for women. It came as something of a shock to me to find that the women as a minority group were completely marginalised by the rest of the hospital.

Most of the therapeutic endeavours were geared towards the majority population, which were men. At this time I had also become conscious of the prejudice that affected the delivery of service to both black men and women in England. There had been repeated racial harassment; and also the murder of a young man in 1975 shook the anti-racist establishment. It took a long time, however, for me to begin to recognise the existence of racism and the way it affected the delivery of service to my patients within the institution. It was my black male patients who began to point out the kind of assumptions that I had made about the kind of care they were receiving and how non-valid my assumptions were in relation to what they were experiencing.

While working with the women it had become obvious to me that they, especially black women, were disproportionately represented in secure hospitals or in prison. As with the men there was a diagnosis of a serious process illness in all of them, especially that of schizophrenia. (Four per cent of the community are black, yet 12% of the women diagnosed as suffering from schizophrenia are black.)

Most research suggested that the higher incidence of schizophrenia was genetically determined. Harrison et al. (1988) suggested a higher incidence of schizophrenia in second generation black people. In such research there was no recognition that young black men were also educationally deprived and had disadvantages built into their employment prospects.

The black men were subjected to racial harassment not only by neighbours but also by establishment figures. It was quite common for black men to be stopped in the streets of London and searched as they were suspected of carrying or pushing drugs. There was also an assumption that they would be unemployed and also that they would be educationally underachieving. The whole black psyche, particularly of the black male, was therefore distorted and damaged.

BROADMOOR HOSPITAL

All these prejudices were reflected in the way black male patients were managed in closed institutions like Broadmoor Hospital.

In risk assessment, 'blackness' was an important factor in assessing patients' future violent behaviour. It was also assumed that the black patient would have substance abuse problems, including using hard drugs, even though it is known that the black community tends to abuse cannabis more than abusing cocaine or morphine. Despite the diagnosis of schizophrenia the black male patient was also perceived as being 'bad'. Seclusion statistics show that there was a tendency to seclude black men before they had committed an act of aggression on the basis that they *were likely to* do so.

Perception of the violent black youngster was further exaggerated and accentuated by the kind of research that was being carried out by the psychiatric establishment. A congregation of black patients on a particular ward was described as black men forming a ghetto so that they could then use the ward to supply drugs.

Within the hospital mentally ill black patients were left on much higher doses of medication for a longer period of time as compared with white male patients with the same symptoms.

On the two male wards where I worked in Broadmoor Hospital there was an increasing recognition, particularly by the nursing staff, that a lot of the black male patients had been exposed to a considerable amount of physical and sometimes sexual abuse. The aggression that the black men showed was a reflection of the kind of violence that they had been subjected to throughout their childhood in care homes and other institutions. There were repeated requests, therefore, particularly from the nursing staff, that the black men should have some exposure to psychotherapy, particularly anger management. However, it took nearly three years before the Broadmoor management were willing to appoint a black male psychotherapist to engage the black men in looking at their anger and their aggression.

Punishments such as seclusion and high doses of medication were seen to be more appropriate than talking therapy and any attempt to introduce such led to the charge of inverted racism against the professionals who were trying to bring some kind of cultural change.

The Royal College of Psychiatrists until the 1990s had continuously failed to acknowledge any racism within the delivery of service to the black patient. However, the formation of the Transcultural Psychiatric Interest Group and continuous criticism and pressure from the black groups outside the institutions eventually led to an acknowledgement that the service being delivered to the black men was not only deficient but at times abusive and exploitative (Royal College of Psychiatrists 1996).

I was amazed at the tolerance and the degree of resilience that my black male patients demonstrated during their stay at Broadmoor Hospital. There were incidents of abuse from staff where they were described as 'niggers' or 'asked to go back to where they had come from'. Reports at case conferences described them as manipulative and devious, and there was constant suspicion that they were involved in trafficking and also of taking drugs despite repeated urine tests which showed that they were clear of cannabis.

A lack of appropriate services in the community meant that they were unable to move on from conditions of high security, even when they had been able to satisfy the Broadmoor establishment, and their own clinical team, that they were now safe to return to the community.

The death of three black men in Broadmoor Hospital following medication and seclusion led to an inquiry which suggested that, although not overt, covert racism and institutional racism did exist within the hospital (Prins *et al.* 1993). My experience was that the prejudice was usually quite overt and that was also the experience of the black patients.

In our attempt to develop a service that was sensitive to the needs of the minority we were constantly criticised for being 'racist' ourselves. Any attempts to focus on a service that was directed towards black men and women were then diverted into, 'Why shouldn't we also develop a service for women and what about those who are disabled?'

The black male patient was also perceived as being sexually disinhibited and exploitative in relation to the women patients. Women patients, particularly white women patients, were actively discouraged by their primary nurses in having a relationship with male black patients because they were seen as 'rapists and sex offenders'. Even when women patients expressed a desire to relate to black male patients because they found them less threatening and less aggressive, they were told it was 'their perverted personalities that led them to be attracted towards these awful black men'.

THE BROADER PICTURE

In a joint document of the Department of Health and Home Office on services for people from black and ethnic minority groups, the following statement was made:

> Issues of race and culture are among the most contentious, challenging and sensitive being considered by this review. Results appear from responses to consultation in the earlier advisory group reports, i.e. Reed's community report on patients with special needs, that they are seen by many as among the most important. (Reed Report)

In a workshop that we organised, which included some of my black patients, it was pointed out to me by the black male patients that, despite clear legislation which existed in the UK which deals with discrimination, they were constantly being discriminated against within the hospital.

There is one clause under section 1.1 of the Race Relations Act 1976 which states that a person discriminates against another if: 'he applies to that other a requirement or condition which he applies or would *apply equally* to persons not of the same racial group as that other' (i.e. people from different racial groups should be treated *differently* but *equally*) (Race Relations Act 1976). In fact the host community applied its own norms of behaviour and achievement to the black community. The failure of black men and women to achieve these norms meant that they were seen as genetically inferior (low IQ, educationally underachieving, criminal, etc.)

This was reflected again and again in the identity problems of a black male patient who even denied his origin in an attempt to be accepted by the white community. The young black male was not only rejected by the host community but he then compounded his problems by rejecting his own identity, including his parents and his family. It was therefore not surprising to find one young black man I saw as an out-patient in East London who poured bleach over himself to make himself become white, so that he would be accepted by the community.

A need to reclaim some kind of racial, sexual identity led to a number of black patients getting involved in a very violent lifestyle which was ultimately self-destructive. Statistics suggest that the highest rate of suicide is now amongst young black men (Royal College of Psychiatrists 1996).

The research that was being carried out particularly by the Royal College of Psychiatrists (of which I was a member) was perceived by the community as abusive and exploitative. Constant attempts to justify the diagnosis of schizophrenia through genetic/biological research that suggested a higher incidence of schizophrenia in the black man in this country were not supported by an extensive study carried out in Jamaica (Hickling 1991). It was also found that the course and outcome of schizophrenia was more favourable in developing rather than developed countries (Jablensky *et al.* 1992). This was contrary to the research findings in this country.

In its *Fourth Biennial Report* the Mental Health Commission commented that 'many professionals seem to lack basic knowledge about the differing needs of ethnic minority communities and to have little real understanding of institutional racism and the effects of cultural differences in the nature of mental disorder' (Mental Health Act Commission 1991).

The black patients' experience in the community was repeated in the care services. Members of the black staff at Broadmoor Hospital, particularly the doctors and the nurses, survived by refusing to acknowledge the existence of racism and how that damaged their relationship with their black patients. During the latter part of my stay in Broadmoor Hospital the existence of prejudice was finally acknowledged and addressed by the managers. A number of black members of staff, including medical staff, then felt able to describe to me their own experience of exploitation and prejudice and what that did to them in terms of their valuing themselves.

The most depressing comment in one of the Mental Health Act Commission reports was the observation that 'black patients tended to regard racist attitudes of staff as a normal experience of institutional life that does not qualify as a matter for complaint' (Mental Health Act Commission 1991). That was also the experience of the black staff in closed institutions.

BLACK WOMEN

In such a climate it is inevitable that all women, but especially black women, will be disproportionately represented in secure hospital or in prison.

Institutions such as marriage and family have been found to be increasingly exploitative of women. The evidence of the sexual abuse of children by parents and the incidence of domestic violence against women by men also suggests that such institutions are just as likely to be exploitative and oppressive as nurturing.

Most first generation immigrants from Third World countries had been used to the extended family. The denigration of the extended family as a pathological structure and the promotion of the nuclear family as the acceptable norm has led to the complete breakdown of the extended 'black family'. This has been especially difficult for the black woman who has now lost any concept of role modelling. The nuclear family has proved to be non-nurturing both to the white and the black community. The black woman, however, has been left with having to manage the black child and also to cope with the displaced anger of the black man who has lost his role within the nuclear family.

The double disadvantage of being black and a woman is reflected in the available statistics. As already stated, a higher percentage of black women than black men are in remand and a higher percentage are diagnosed as suffering from mental disorder. (Black women on remand – drug couriers from Third World countries). (Home Office Statistics)

Women are more likely than men to receive a psychiatric referral as a result of a criminal charge. Women also get admitted to secure facilities for less serious offences than men and once admitted usually spend longer in such hospitals. This becomes understandable when one looks at the therapy that is being offered to women. Concepts such as normalisation, integration and rehabilitation, which became popular in the 1960s, are still being adhered to without any acknowledgement of the changing nature of society and its institution. The concept of gender role *normalism* continues to promote men and women as having differing social roles which are biologically determined.

The nurturing role of the woman and the provider role of the man are still enshrined in therapy. For the black woman who has suffered double exploitation such normalism is totally alienating. Most black women find it extremely difficult to internalise the concept of normal behaviour as dictated by a predominantly white male community. Most Third World women have grown up in a predominantly 'women culture' and they have coped with the male ethos of the society that they live in by developing defense mechanisms which are peculiar to themselves. For example, most black women grow up in a home that is managed by the mother and the grandmother.

There are clear role models in terms of the girl child, and the specification of the roles allows a certain amount of confidence in terms of their identity that is not available in white male-dominated British society. In institutions such as Broadmoor the promotion of these norms is particularly difficult for the black woman patient. Most black women cope with such situations by withdrawing into themselves. The black woman is then described as arrogant, aggressive and manipulative.

Since most of these women have been abused within a heterosexual nuclear family, therapeutic endeavours directed towards institutional normalisation of this kind becomes a bizarre, alienating and in fact abusive process for them.

GENDER INTEGRATION

Gender *integration* is another such hallowed concept, which was enthusiastically promoted in the 1960s to reduce institutionalisation. During the 1970s and 1980s integration of patients' living areas has continued without any acceptance of the concept of sexual liberation that was associated with it in the 1960s. In fact, the moral climate from the 1970s to date has been towards promotion of Victorian values in relation to sexual behaviour.

We are therefore now in the absurd situation of expecting our women patients to live in close proximity to totally strange men in what is promoted as having to be an asexual environment (a therapeutic environment) and promoting this as a process of normalisation. This is particularly difficult for black women who have no experience of such 'heterosexual norms'.

Despite repeated allegations of rape by women patients, committed against them by male patients and sometimes by male staff, integrated wards continue to remain within psychiatric units. The double jeopardy of being a black woman and also being labelled mentally disordered means that the woman patient is seldom believed anyway.

REHABILITATION

In the 1960s *rehabilitation* of the mentally disordered patient became an essential part of the patient's treatment. This was in the era of de-institutionalisation. Rehabilitation in the 1960s and into the 1970s was therefore about the empowering of the individual and for him or her to be able to operate in his/her own environment. Rehabilitation, choice, empowerment were therefore built into the overall ideology of equality of opportunity for all.

Through the 1980s and 1990s, however, de-institutionalisation has become synonymous with cheap after-care. Institutions have been closed without appropriate funding in the community and patients have been turned out of large Victorian wards in rural surroundings to live in small flats in the inner cities.

The breaking down of the extended family has led to black women feeling isolated and marginalised and any hospitalisation has meant the loss of her children. Black women patients who have been incarcerated have had their children taken into care and are usually refused access. Very few family units exist that would allow a mentally ill mother to remain with her children and be treated during the acute phase of her illness. There are no mother and baby units for black women only. Current statistics regarding the increase of black children in care reflect the failure of the psychiatric services to appropriately look after such women and their children (Social Services Reports).

Rehabilitation within the institution or in the community continues to emphasise individual responsibility without in any way empowering the person. The woman patient is therefore subjected to continuous double messages that hold her responsible for social inadequacies over which she not only has no control but of which she herself is a victim.

The black community has therefore become more and more alienated from a service that still promotes therapy but which is now anti-therapeutic.

CONCLUSION

It is my opinion that we will not address the feelings of alienation and rejection of our black patients unless we recognise the deficiency within the services.

I believe we need to continue to validate our patients' experiences instead of denying them or labelling them as pathological. We also need to recognise that many of our institutions such as family and marriage have been abusive and exploitative of our black patients, particularly the black women.

The responsibility needs also to be shifted to where it belongs (which is the responsibility of the entire society to manage an individual who is disordered and distressed) and not hold the individual responsible for their illness.

We need to be aware that some of our hallowed concepts in terms of therapy in fact are abusive and exploitative and cannot be therapeutic.

In relation to the black community we need to recognise that our prejudices have affected the delivery of care and that this has diminished both them and us in the process.

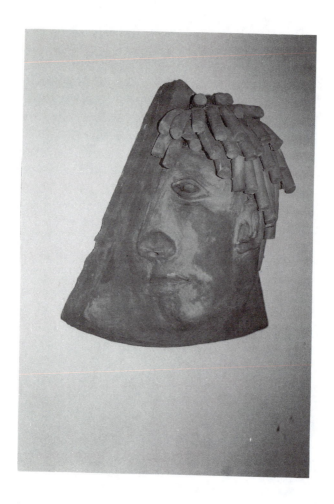

'Profile'. Clay Tablet – David

CHAPTER 11

Black Men in Broadmoor

Stan Grant

As a therapist the challenge for me is not only having to work with the material that the patients present but also the material that the institution of psychiatry and the institution of Broadmoor presents.

ANOTHER COUNTRY

As I wander down these your dusty roads
I wonder what are the different codes
That you live by
The different codes that you live by
I wonder when you look at me just
What it is that you see
With your trained eye
That you see with your trained eye
Like me is it the same for you
Hard to see through the things you do
To the real you
The things you do to the real you
Each one has to find a way of living
Each one navigates the world that they know
So tell me just what it is we should be giving
When our two worlds meet which way do we go
I thought I knew the meaning of what
Is my world
Now I'm in yours I have to question mine
I'm in yours I have to question mine
But am I really in this world that
You call yours or
Peeping in from the outside
Just peeping in from the outside
So where do we go to really find the meaning?

What can we hold on to that we know is true?
Must I keep on wondering how you see me?
Must I tell you what I see when I see you
As I wander down these your dusty roads
I wonder what are the different codes
That you live by
The different codes that you live by

(Lyric copyright: Arike aka Stan Grant)

WHY A BLACK THERAPIST?

The discussion of black men in Broadmoor is of necessity a political discussion which must make reference to the history of psychiatry and the impact of racism. When we use the word 'black' we are automatically tapping in to a whole stream of connotations that exist in the European psyche both conscious and unconscious. Historically for Europeans black is seen as negative, evil, darkness, the unknown, bad, damned, dirty, away from the light. Black people have been perceived as primitive, uneducated, stupid, dirty, evil, ungodly, heathen, animalistic, non-human, inferior, cannibals, the sexual, exploitable, expendable, simple, lazy, immoral, irresponsible and much more. Currently in this society additional stereotypes abound about black people as trouble-makers, anti-authority, muggers, violent, rapists and scroungers.

I am not writing from a neutral and detached position – I am being deliberately subjective. I am writing as a black man born in this country fifty years ago, into a white supremacist society. I am writing as a man whose father was diagnosed as schizophrenic by the mental health system, taken from him and never seen again. I am writing from the position of an educated black man who has been described as 'well-adjusted' and who recognises the loss that this *acculturation* has meant.

Other contributors to this book have written extensively elsewhere on the issues of 'race, ' 'culture' and psychiatry, and these works provide an in-depth backdrop to the issues briefly touched on here. What follows are some reflections, some reflections on a beginning. This beginning has been about fourteen months in the making and it is still ongoing. At some point we will have moved beyond this stage and then there will be another story to tell. For the time being, however, the focus is on getting started.

The hospital authority is to be applauded for the insight and determination of some of its staff members, namely the Equal Opportunities Working Group, in recognising a need and pressing for the inclusion of a black therapist amongst its staff, which has resulted in my appointment. The responses to my being in the hospital have been varied: 'We can learn a lot from you, ' 'You must let us know what you do, ' 'Tell us where we are getting it wrong, ' 'Surely this is divisive!' and the most telling has been, 'Why do you need a black therapist, surely it's just the same?' I have been in the post for just over a year now and, judging by recent conversations, this latter view is still intact.

In its political correctness the authority has admitted that there is the possibility that it might be complicit in perpetuating the mistreatment of a particular group within the hospital and has thus sanctioned the appointment, but it seems that it has yet to be convinced of its value.

We must consider the setting for this work. Broadmoor is not a 'regular' prison and neither is it a 'regular' hospital. It is a hospital for the mentally disordered offender. What this means is that the men are incarcerated for having committed crimes whilst, in society's eyes, being of unsound mind, mentally disordered. So in addition to the incarceration for their offence, they must take part in a programme designed to address the 'soundness,' or its lack, of their mind. In the 'outside' world the relationship of the therapist with an individual or group would be determined by that individual or group with the therapist. However, in this situation there are other agendas and this puts the role of the therapist into question. Who am I working with? Who am I working for? What is the aim? Whose agenda is followed?

What is my work with these black men? What is it that the role demands of me that will enable me to be a useful resource for the men that decide to take advantage of the group? What is my model of working? How has my training equipped me to deal with the particular situation of working with black men in Broadmoor?

I am clear that my role is not determined by the 'forensic' agenda of the institution. Inevitably I am invited to give reports on the men that I work with that are used in a forensic context; however, my prime focus is on the men and their personal development. For some of the men they may not see that distinction, and will link my work with them to a potential earlier release. They will be participating in the group with that aim in mind. This may be a possible outcome of their work with me, but for me my concern has to do with the men's insight into and understanding of their own behaviour, perceptions and beliefs that will enable them to make more informed pro-survival choices and take charge of their lives.

In a society that the black man perceives as unjust, a society that perceives him with negative regard, the black man will use whatever means necessary to survive. These means would be very different were the society to respect him and regard him in the same light as his white counterpart. Whilst in no way condoning some of the 'survival' behaviours that these men engage in, I see them as understandable. The work I have as a therapist then is thus quite complex. I see it as assisting these men to regain a sense of pride and dignity in themselves, these men whom the society holds in contempt, enabling them to make choices that are pro-survival, i.e. respectful of both themselves and others, that damage neither themselves nor others.

My formal training has given me a 'basic' understanding of human development, human processes and human functioning. But the particular elements that we have in this situation, so-called mentally disordered offenders in a white dominated institution in a white supremacist society, cannot be understood from within the narrow framework of the Eurocentric training that I received. I need to make reference elsewhere, to other disciplines and to my own experience. This is not about re-inventing the wheel but about a recognition that I am exploring uncharted territory. I have in the past run groups for black men, but this has been on 'the outside' where the men attended voluntarily and had a certain degree of willingness and commitment to explore their situation. I am not implying that the men in Broadmoor are not willing, but the men on the outside had their liberty and could ultimately determine the level of their engagement without any pressure or coercion to engage in a particular way, and could choose to leave if they so wished.

My personal practice of Re-evaluation Counselling has given me a way to think about my own life and theorise about us as humans. It is my belief that, barring damage to our brains or mental apparatus, we are all able to function well in all circumstances. The extent to which we do not bears a direct relation to those times in our lives when we have been hurt, mistreated or oppressed in some way resulting in us being unable to make sense of, heal, resolve or assimilate what was happening to us at the time. These distress experiences are painful to us and we make an unconscious decision each time they happen to try and work it through at some later stage, to clean it up and be healed from it.

If we, by good fortune, get an opportunity to do this, the memory of the original situation is stored as a memory from which we learn but with no painful emotion attached. The chances are, however, that that which led to lack of resolution, lack of understanding and lack of healing in the first place will be replicated later. I am talking here about the attention of an aware person who understands the importance of emotional discharge and who is able to support another to do this.

This emotional discharge is the process that we need to go through to make sense of, heal, resolve and free ourselves from the effects of our past distress experiences and is characterised by crying, laughing, yawning, trembling, raging and so on. The absence of this support at the time of a distress experience leaves us with a rigid patterned behaviour and way of feeling that obscures our usual effective functioning. When we act from that rigid, patterned place we tend to behave in ways that are anti-survival, i.e. not in the best interests of ourselves or other people, and much damage can be done.

These are the principles from which I operate in my own personal therapeutic process and I try to incorporate them into my professional work. Thus my aim as a therapist is to enable the persons that I work with to work through their unresolved hurts and free themselves from the rigid behaviour that this leaves them with and thus return to full functioning. Trying to do this at Broadmoor has been a major challenge. I want here, using various quotes, to provide a sketch backdrop and context within which to understand the work.

THE PROBLEM OF PREJUDICE AND POWER

We are all products of our upbringing, our histories and our education. Our ideas, values and perspectives get handed down from generation to generation much as tradition and myth, stereotype and misinformation. The legacy of this is what we have today – unequal positions in society of white people and black people. Broadmoor is an institution which is based on psychiatry, but what kind of psychiatry is it? Is it objective? Is it unbiased? What myths, stereotypes and misinformation inform its practice?

Fernando (1991, p.115) observes that: 'When racism does occur – its presence is seldom acknowledged. Hence questions about racism in British psychiatry are not being faced openly.' Greenwood (1995) states that:

In psychiatry, as the rules of diagnosis are usually made by White Western psychiatrists, the norms, the socially acceptable behaviours against which they test their clients, are the norms of White Western society. Thus appearance, demeanour, behaviour, attitudes, beliefs, thoughts and feelings or their particular combinations are defined as 'sick', 'psychotic', 'mad', 'abnormal' or 'disturbed' if they differ in certain ways from whatever is regarded as normal in today's White society in the countries of the Western World.

The cultural perceptions that we see manifest in the society's institutions today have a direct link to the attitudes and beliefs that were prevalent in earlier times. Peter Fryer (1993, p.28), who asserts that 'racist ideology sprang from slavery', provides many illustrations that enable us to trace this ideology to the present day:

Every planter knows that there are negroes, who ... cannot be humanised as others are, that they will remain with respect to their understanding, but a few degrees removed from the ourang outang (i.e. the chimpanzee and gorilla); and from which many negroes may be supposed, without any very improbable conjecture[,] to be the offspring. (John Gardner, Jamaica planter, 1783, quoted in Fryer 1993, p.27)

We have a population to deal with [in the British West Indies], the enormous majority of whom are of an inferior race ... Give them independence, and in a few generations they will peel off such civilisation as they have learnt as easily and willingly as their coats and trousers. (James Anthony Froude, Regius Professor of Modern History at Oxford, 1888, quoted in Fryer 1993, p.37)

In 1956 Churchill's Cabinet, concerned about a 'coloured invasion', asked for information from the Metropolitan Police and staffs of labour exchanges. The Metropolitan Police reported that:

> on the whole coloured people are work-shy and content to live on national assistance and immoral earnings. They are poor workmen ... They are said to be of low mentality and will only work for short periods. (Fryer 1993)

Fryer also goes on to say that:

> We had not long ago a Metropolitan Police commissioner who told an American journalist that 'in the Jamaicans, you have a people who are constitutionally disorderly ... It's simply in their make-up. They are constitutionally disposed to be anti-authority.'

It is not such a great leap from this to MIND's (1993) observation that:

> Much research about black and minority ethnic people and mental health locates the 'problem' or 'schizophrenia' either in their genes or their culture and does not pay sufficient attention to the impact of racism outside and in the mental health system.

Browne (1995) in his research into the impact that the race (of the prospective patient) might have on decision-making involved in the application of the civil sections of the Mental Health Act notes the following view from one of the 14 police officers interviewed:

> If you can't understand them then they probably won't be able to understand you therefore the more likely you are to find yourself using some form of restraint. Violence is more of a factor because persuasion can't be used – and particular [racial] groups tend to be more excitable than others.

Ponterotto and Pedersen (1993, p.18) have said whilst discussing prejudice:

> One major theme pervading the newer conceptions of prejudice is that racist attitudes and beliefs are outside conscious awareness. Given that racist views contradict most people's stated value system, one's view of self would be impacted negatively if a racist ideology were acknowledged. Therefore, holding racist beliefs out of conscious awareness keeps the self-concept intact.

They continue, asserting that:

> It is natural for people to cling to their own values and personal views and to hold them in high esteem. It is also common for people to prefer their own 'in group' – family, religious group, ethnic group – to 'out groups'. (p.27)

They add, whilst referring to Allport (1979), *The Nature of Prejudice*:

Often, however, and without sufficient warrant, people exaggerate the virtues of their own group. Allport uses the term 'love prejudice' to refer to people's tendency to overgeneralise the virtues of their own values, family, and group. Love prejudice toward one's own group can lead towards antagonism towards outside groups, and thus serve as the foundation for ethnocentrism. Aboud (1987, p.49, 'The development of ethnic self-identification and attitudes') defines ethnocentrism as 'an exaggerated preference for one's group and concomitant dislike of other groups'. Ethnocentrism serves as a building block for negative racial prejudice (Ponterotto 1991).

MP Paul Boateng has said that the mental health care system is 'very dangerous for young black people to get involved with' (Boateng 1997). This is consistent with MIND's assertions (MIND 1993). In its *Policy on Black and Minority Ethnic People and Mental Health* it states: 'Racism can damage people's mental health and racism in mental health services often compounds distress.'

In providing a context for this assertion MIND notes that studies over the past 20 years show:

- Black people are more likely than white to be:
  - removed by the police to a place of safety under section 136 of the Mental Health Act 1983
  - detained in hospital under sections 2, 3, and 4 of the Mental Health Act
  - diagnosed as suffering from schizophrenia or another form of psychotic illness
  - detained in locked wards of psychiatric hospitals
  - given higher doses of medication.
- Black people are less likely than white people to:
  - receive appropriate and acceptable diagnosis or treatment for possible
  - mental illness' at an early stage
  - receive treatments such as psychotherapy or counselling.

Users' observations and experiences of the mental health system add another dimension to this illustration:

Racist behaviour is most frequently meted out by local staff who receive little training, and bring all their prejudices to the workplace from the community in which they live. (Veronica Dewan, ex-service-user, 1996)

I mean, although slavery was legally abolished in the eighteen hundreds, racism still continues. It is a wound that remains today in the soul of many 'blacks', propelling a growing percentage of young black men towards violence. We neither understand our actions nor can we find a way out from the shroud of death which broods over our neighbourhoods throughout the world. The fact is, much of the violence in our cities today is the bitter fruit of a tree that the white race cultivated in racism. (Broadmoor patient 1997)

There were about 8 or 10 of them, all on top of me holding me down. I was big then, about 16 and a half stone. Its the drugs, they have that effect – bloat you up. So they're on top of me and I suddenly realised, 'This is it!' they're gonna kill me – I'm gonna become a statistic. So I thought there's no way they're gonna take me out without me taking one of them. He had his arm round my throat, squeezing tighter – I couldn't breathe – I asked him to stop – he wouldn't. So it was a death grip – do you know what that is? I was fighting for my life and I found this surge of strength – I grabbed her neck and squeezed – she was starting to go cyanose, I was too but on a black person they couldn't tell – try as they might to remove my hands they just could not. It was either her life or mine – they let go. I'm in no doubt whatsoever that had I not done that I would be dead now. (Broadmoor patient 1997)

You can't trust these people – they are a law unto themselves – they get away with murder here. If for any reason you cross them, they don't like you or they see you as a problem, all they've got to do is put it down on paper and it's on your record. It doesn't matter that it's not true, when another colleague reads it then to them it is true, and so on it goes. It's only your word against theirs and you know who is going to be believed. (Broadmoor patient 1997)

When a person is not acknowledged he loses his spirit ... In the more severe cases, lack of acknowledgement and lack of spirit will manifest in Black men as confusion, hopelessness, and disrespect for life and other living things. (Vanzant 1996)

GETTING STARTED

Ultimately each person must take responsibility for how they behave – external forces must not be used as an excuse to evade this. However, external forces do impinge on how a person perceives, thinks, makes decisions, acts and feels. The work of the group has to take account of both the external and internal forces operating on a person in order to gain clarity about appropriate behaviour. Like those from other groups a fundamental desire for black people is to be and be seen as being a fully-fledged member of the 'human group'. This leaves the black person living in a white supremacist society in a dilemma. On the one hand he or she wants to be a part of society and on the other hand they are made to feel apart from it.

There are men in the group who see benefit for themselves in attending. However, as a result of comments picked up from some of the men I am forced to ask: to what extent does the fact they are required to attend the group as part of their care militate against its therapeutic value? Some of the possible dynamics that this can set up are:

- therapy is seen as a burden, something to be endured in order to fulfil the requirements
- lack of willingness to engage
- subversion of the process
- therapy seen as something that is done to them
- therapy as punitive, as a stick to beat them, as one more weapon that is used to manipulate them into conformity
- 'us' and 'them' polarity
- mistrust.

The men in the therapy group are at different stages of development, and because there are differences in terms of perspectives the potential is always present for tense and difficult interpersonal dynamics in the group.

There is progress but it is slow. Before my appointment at Broadmoor a therapist of African heritage had not been available for the males of African heritage who are patients there. On my arrival I was told by some of the patients, in a matter-of-fact way that disguised both anger and disappointment, that I was three and a half years too late. For these particular men they had drawn on their own resources in the interim and had done whatever work was needed for themselves by themselves. However, they felt that since they had made such a fuss about having a black therapist and at long last it had materialised in the appointment of myself, then rather than risk losing the opportunity they must support it for the benefit of others, even though they had made advances in their own personal development unassisted. They were uncertain about the benefits to themselves and adopted an attitude of watch and see.

The candidates for the group were men who had primarily been identified by Chandra Ghosh, who together with the Equal Opportunities Working Group has been the driving force in bringing the group into existence. They were unprepared and uncertain about the group, had not met with me, and I think curiosity played a large part for them in coming, nothing quite like this ever having existed before. The group eventually began, had a life of about ten weeks and has never re-formed. Since that time, whilst seeing men individually, I have been attempting to restart the group in a way that is more appropriate. By this I mean where I have had an opportunity to meet with each man, to talk with him about my ideas and the potential for such a project, for him to have the opportunity to ask any questions of me and clarify for himself if the group is something that he might want to participate in. This has not been easy, since the time that I have at the hospital is patient contact time, and so doing the necessary groundwork has been hampered by lack of time.

I sought and won approval for a second therapist to join me and at the time of writing that person, Clifford Henry, has just begun, in a voluntary capacity, with a view to eventually being engaged as a professional. At the same time I also sought and won approval for an increase in hours so that I could do the necessary development work to support and sustain the group. It was agreed in principle but would have to wait for funding until the new financial year. At present Cliff and I are interviewing men for the new group. Whilst this has been going on the hospital has had difficulty in finding a suitable venue for the group and resolving the issue of how the necessary escorts will be funded. So after just over a year of being in the institution it feels as if we are just beginning. The life of the original group was short-lived but I want to share with you some of the thoughts arising out of this experience.

I came to be invited to work as a therapist in Broadmoor as a result of having been called in to cover a training session for Luke Daniels who was unavailable to do it. In order to check my suitability for this session I was invited to submit my CV. It was then noticed that I might fit the bill for a therapy group for black men that was being mooted. I was invited to consider this and was interviewed and accepted for the post. The impetus for this had come from the Equal Opportunities Working Group. I do not know about the evolution of this idea from an institutional and management perspective but my suspicion is that it has not been easy gaining acceptance of the idea of a black therapist for black patients. The resistance to the idea and reluctance to accept its usefulness has been tangible ever since my arrival. The Equal Opportunities Working Group, which funds my post, has a limited budget, with competing bids for a slice of it. In the long term it would make sense for the post to be funded from the mainstream budget, but I am wary of this until a greater acceptance is demonstrated for the existence of the idea of black-on-black therapy.

That the hospital is also unclear as to how to nurture and develop this project is evidenced by my entrance into the post. Broadmoor has a very thorough programme of induction that enables each new employee to adjust to being in the hospital. One becomes aware of the ethos of the institution and has instilled in them the importance of safety and security. What is covered is the minimum to enable a person to conduct themselves appropriately on site. This is at a general level and I have appreciated this; however, I have had no further induction to support me to successfully carry out my role. I have turned to Chandra Ghosh, who, sadly for me, is no longer at the hospital, and Tony Lingiah as my key support people in attempting to come to terms with the reality of Broadmoor. On a practical level John King has been my main support in trying to move things forward to get the new group started. At present the structure does not exist on a practical level for me to tap into the support that could be enjoyed from the rest of the therapeutic community in Broadmoor. One might be tempted to say that this is purely down to budgetary considerations but the pragmatist in me believes that it is an issue of will.

THE SHORT LIFE OF THE FIRST GROUP

I inherited a group of men who I had never met before and none of whom had been prepared for this group. I was met with equal doses of curiosity and suspicion: 'Who is this man with black skin holding keys?' There is a derogatory term that is used within the black community to refer to someone who has a black skin but whose consciousness separates them from their black identity. This term is 'coconut' and some of the staff at Broadmoor are perceived in this way. 'Is he to be trusted?', 'Why is he in this role carrying keys?', 'Is he a coconut?', 'What kind of black man is he – look how he dresses – look how he talks!', 'What does he know about the street?', 'Is he going to come with all them white man's theories to try to get in my head?', 'What's in it for him?', 'Why is he here now?', 'Why just black men – there's nothing he can tell me about being black – what does he know?'

The role of a therapist, like that of a doctor or lawyer, is based on a relationship of confidentiality with the patient. One would suspect that in an institution such as Broadmoor there would need to be some discussion with the care team and management as to what in practical terms this means. To date this discussion has yet to take place. In the absence of a clearly stated agenda from the institution, I am left to my own devices. My agenda with the men is a personal developmental one whereby they are afforded time and space to reflect on themselves and take stock of their situation. In that process they get to consider whether they want or need to make any changes, and they determine for themselves whether to initiate such changes. On starting the group it was clear that for a number of men, if not all of them, their primary concern was: 'How is this going to help me get out of here?'

The attendance of the group fluctuated – at its peak there were seven men attending, but it averaged around four. Although other men in the group gave their perceptions and opinions, not having time other than direct contact time I was unable, with certainty, to ascertain the reasons for the fluctuations. Undoubtedly a contributing factor has been the removal from the ward of some of the men as a consequence of skirmishes and fights with other patients. We can also assume that some of it must have been to do with the issues of a group in its forming stages. As mentioned above most of the men were concerned to know to what extent participating in the group was going to contribute to their early release. Having explained my perception of the group's purpose as outlined above I lost men.

The earlier sessions concentrated on exploring and laying down the boundaries for the group's operation and dealt with issues of how we would treat one another. Frictions and tensions existed in the men's relationships with one another prior to the group's start, and these became magnified at this beginning stage. For some of the men, even though the group was still forming, they saw it as being unable to contain or manage these tensions. This was despite the work done on ground-rules and setting the tone of the group.

In the wide world members of a therapy group can come together for the duration of the group's meeting and leave when the session ends. For these men no such option exists – they are on the same ward and have nowhere to go. As a result they are, understandably, very guarded and give very little in order to ensure their own safety. Their uncertainty about me and their uncertainty about each other in this context means that trying to establish a basis of rapport is fraught with difficulty.

The focus in the early days is on the outer rather than the inner, on the state of the world, on 'the system', on Broadmoor, on racism. All of these, however, are essential and key components in the work to be done; they provide a framework and context for understanding the men's relationship to the dominant society and its systems. At the same time this strategy is used as a way of distancing themselves from me and from each other. It is a legitimate way of communicating thoughts and feelings about their situation and allows them to feel righteous indignation without showing much of themselves. This strategy is also used as a way to get the measure of me, to see 'where I'm coming from' and to begin to check out the boundaries of the process.

Eventually they manage to reflect and think about themselves and each other. They are able to own that there is room for change in themselves and talk about this. They are able to offer feedback to each other which is positive and most, though unused to this, find it pleasing. The following week they found it hard to remember what was said and so we went through the process again with people this time identifying what they wanted to change. At this point they took the opportunity to give me feedback. I was told that I am too optimistic and that I am somewhat naïve about what it is like for them as black men in Broadmoor. I was told that the racism is real and that I would have to live their experience to really see what goes on. Some of the men, in their terms, perceive themselves as mentally healthy and that being among 'mentally ill' people has a negative impact on them.

For the reasons outlined above the group eventually ceased to function as a group and I began to see people individually. Currently my new colleague, Cliff, and I have been interviewing the men in preparation for a new group. We have seen most of them once and we are about to embark on our second visit. Provided that the escorting and venue get sorted out, we will be up and running in the spring.

CHAPTER 12

Providing Clinical Care for Black Patients in Forensic Psychiatry

Harvey Gordon

RACE AND PSYCHIATRY

Britain has an ethnically diverse population and one of the largest ethnic minorities in Britain is the West Indian community, consisting of black people born in the West Indies or whose parents were born there. Most of those are from Jamaica, but lesser numbers come from other islands such as Trinidad, St Lucia and Grenada. Those of West Indian origin significantly outnumber the black African population in Britain (Nazroo 1997). However, the term African-Caribbean is often used to denote linkage between black Africans and black Caribbeans. Although historically they have a common African origin, in contemporary British society, whilst they share the same colour of skin, they have a diversity of culture, religion and social development (Hutchinson and McKenzie 1995).

The history of the black population in Western Europe and North America is one of serial forms of victimisation by abduction, transportation, slavery, racial discrimination and race hatred over the last three hundred years. Concurrently, however, the movements to counter such practice have also been prominent. The abolition of slavery by Britain and subsequently by the United States can be seen as stages towards human freedom and equality of opportunity. The struggle against racial discrimination continues to be actively pursued in Western societies. Nonetheless, the transgenerational effects of racism leave their mark (Comer 1985; Marger 1991) and black people can with rationality retain a degree of suspicion about the attitudes of the white majority.

The history of psychiatry is not beyond criticism in regard to its conceptions of ethnic minorities (Bhopal 1997). European and North American culture were seen as superior to the primitive or savage mentality of the black population (Fernando 1991). Some argued that the black person was relatively free of insanity whilst subject to slavery, but became prey to mental disturbance when set free (Thomas and Sillen 1972). Psychiatrists have also separately contributed to ethnically prejudicial perspectives in regard to French colonial oppression of Algeria (Begue 1996; Verges 1996) and the aberrant practices during the Nazi period towards the Jewish and gypsy population (Burleigh 1997; Hanauske-Abel 1996; Lifton 1982).

SCHIZOPHRENIA

The major mental illness of schizophrenia is generally regarded as evenly distributed nationally across the world. The International Pilot Study on Schizophrenia (World Health Organisation 1973, 1979) conducted in nine centres, Aarhus in Denmark, Agra in India, Cali in Columbia, Ibadan in Nigeria, London in England, Moscow in the former Soviet Union, Prague in the Czech Republic, Taipei in Taiwan and Washington in the United States, had shown uniform rates, except for the United States and the former Soviet Union, in both of which rates were elevated due essentially to variations in diagnostic criteria (Cooper et al. 1972; Reich 1991; Smith 1986).

Although the West Indies was not one of the centres researched by the International Pilot Study, other studies have not revealed any notable differences in prevalence of schizophrenia in those islands (Bhugra et al. 1996; Hickling 1991; Hickling and Rodgers-Johnson 1995).

Higher than expected rates of schizophrenia among Caribbean-born people in Britain were however first noted in the 1960s (Hemsi 1967). Subsequent studies of hospital admissions for schizophrenia have consistently reported rates in the African-Caribbean community of ten or more times that of the general population (Harrison et al. 1988), constituting what might be termed an epidemic (Sugarman and Crauford 1994). The highest rates have been found in second generation young male adults of African-Caribbean origin (Glover 1989; Harrison et al. 1997; McGovern and Cope 1987a). These findings have been variously contested on the grounds that schizophrenia is being misdiagnosed in the black population (Sashidharan 1993), whilst one study by Nazroo (1997) failed to replicate the previously grossly elevated rates in African-Caribbeans.

Other studies have shown that African-Caribbeans are over-represented amongst offender patients (McGovern and Cope 1987b; Walker and McCabe 1973); more likely to be admitted to locked wards in general psychiatric hospitals (Bolton 1984; Moodley and Thornicroft 1988); more likely to be admitted to medium secure units (Bullard and Bond 1988; Cope and Ndegwa 1990; Mohan et al. 1997; Shetty and Higgo 1987) and to special hospitals (Coldwell and Naismith 1989; Taylor et al. 1998). It is of note that the excess of African-Caribbeans admitted to special hospitals pertains to those with a diagnosis of psychosis and there is under-representation in regard to the legal category of Psychopathic Disorder (Coid 1992; Shubsachs *et al.* 1995; Taylor *et al.* 1998). Those who are disinclined to the view that any psychopath should be admitted compulsorily to special hospitals (Chiswick 1992; Grounds 1987) may express relief at such a finding, whereas others who feel there is a role for such admissions in selected cases (Coid 1992; Gordon 1996; Gunn 1992; Hamilton 1987; Reiss, Grubin and Meux 1996) may see such under-representation as a paradoxical form of negative discrimination towards the black population!!

SPECIAL HOSPITALS

During the last two decades, the special hospitals have been the subject of extensive professional and public criticism (Department of Health 1992; Department of Health and Social Security 1980; Prins *et al.* 1993).

In regard to the black community, serious unease developed following the deaths in Broadmoor Hospital of three young black male patients between 1984 and 1991 (Prins *et al.* 1993; Ritchie 1985; Special Hospitals Service Authority 1989). Deaths of black people in police custody have further fuelled the apprehension of the black community (Jasper 1998).

In the context of the special hospitals being seen as in need of reform or even abolition, and more specifically the black community perceiving them as institutions in which black patients have died, a degree of considerable mistrust has developed in regard to the capability of the special hospitals to understand and effectively and safely treat the black patient. Special hospitals are seen by many black people as part of the oppressive machinery of society: part of the same system as prisons and the criminal justice system. The principal remit of special hospitals is to afford treatment to mentally disordered patients who pose a serious danger to the public. However, it is at times the patients them-selves and their families who now perceive the danger as coming from the mental health system directed to the black community (Brindle 1997). Black patients have sometimes claimed that patients of African-Caribbean origin in Broadmoor Hospital were killed and not just that they died by unintended error.

There were indeed a range of common factors which pertained to the deaths of the three black patients who died in Broadmoor Hospital between 1984 and 1991. All three were African-Caribbean and all three died after an episode of behavioural disturbance resulting in their being secluded and then given medication without their consent. All three were young black men who had been diagnosed as suffering from a chronic schizophrenic illness, at least by some psychiatrists. All three showed limited insight into their illness and had a history of violence to others associated with their psychoses. Two of the three patients died in the male special care unit for the most disturbed male patients in the hospital, whilst the other died in an ordinary ward, and all three died within a minute or so of having been medicated without their consent.

The deaths of these three black men is a tragedy for the patients themselves, their families and the communities from which they come, for all of whom their grief has been painful in the extreme. Allegations of racism, or at least of racial insensitivity or lack of racial awareness having played a role, were reflected in the Inquiry Report (Prins *et al.* 1993) and by subsequent commentaries (Lipsedge 1994) and resound still today (Fernando, Ndegwa and Wilson 1998).

However, it is far from evident that the deaths of any of the three black patients who died in Broadmoor Hospital were related to racially discriminatory practices. Sudden unexpected deaths of psychiatric patients occurred before neuroleptic medication was available (Davis and Zhang 1988) and are known to occur across the world (Mehtonen *et al.* 1991; Simpson *et al.* 1988) as indeed are sudden deaths in people not known to be suffering from any physical or psychiatric illness at all (Brown and Kocsis 1984; Weatherall, Ledingham and Warrell 1996). Tranquillisation of disturbed psychiatric patients in hospital is common (Hillam and Evans 1996; Pilowsky *et al.* 1992; Simpson and Anderson 1996), yet sudden death or serious adverse reactions are relatively uncommon. Mortality rates are also known to be higher in patients with schizophrenia compared with the general population (Harris and Barraclough 1998). Death following agitation and over-arousal may also be relevant in some cases (Farnham and Kennedy 1997). There is also some evidence of racial differences in rates of various physical illnesses such as diabetes as well possibly in responses to medication (Allen, Rack and Vaddadi 1977; Lewis *et al.* 1980; Marmot, Adelstein and Bulusu 1984). There are therefore many factors that may have collided and contributed to these three deaths without politicising the cause to one related to racism. This is not in any way to imply that all is perfect at Broadmoor or any other hospital in regard to the full appreciation of parameters of healthcare affecting different ethnic groups. It is, however, to suggest that whilst healthcare occurs in a political context, healthcare and politics are not the same phenomena.

THE PSYCHIATRIST'S ROLE TODAY

What then could the individual psychiatrist or health professional do to maximise his or her contribution to the improvement in the mental and physical health of patients of African-Caribbean origin in forensic psychiatry? The psychiatrist should familiarise him/herself with the totality of factors pertaining to the patient, including those of cultural, familial, religious and biological relevance. It is vital to reach an accurate diagnosis or diagnostic formulation in order to afford and monitor the appropriate treatment. An aversion to the diagnosis of schizophrenia or a related psychosis by some psychiatrists, albeit even if they are committed to the improvement of mental healthcare for the black population, may nonetheless be a disservice to those they want to help. A similar aversion to the use, where appropriate, of depot anti-psychotic medication may also be misguided, given the difficulties in ensuring compliance in patients with an illness into which they may show limited or no insight (Buchanan 1998). Untreated or under-treated schizophrenia is a disease with dangers to the patient him/herself and to others and little is achieved by underestimating the severity of the condition. I would speculate that from inquiries held into homicides by psychiatric patients, there are few if any cases where such an incident has been perpetrated by a patient known to have been adequately medicated at the time of the homicide (Howlett 1998). Depression may well be part of the psychotic illness and should be actively and vigorously treated, but should be undertaken concurrently with the treatment of the psychosis, and not by revising the diagnosis from schizophrenia to depression.

Individual or group psychotherapy can also be an important part of the treatment to address issues in the lives of patients causing conflict and which may have been dealt with by the patients in a maladaptive way. Indeed, there is some evidence that black patients are under-represented in those accepted for psychotherapy (Campling 1989).

The identity of the patient as a full and equal human being needs to be emphasised, including where appropriate that being black has been an identity of minority status which has been subject to abuse and discrimination. The psychiatrist should therefore play his/her role in ensuring fair, equal and appropriate treatment for all patients irrespective of colour in the hospital and in the community more widely.

The psychiatrist must, above all, seek to understand his/her own limitations and prejudices, but he/she must also be aware of his/her training, knowledge and experience and dedication to the health of his/her patient.

CHAPTER 13

Black Staff and their Experience at Work

Krishnan Gnanasekaran

INTRODUCTION

It is striking that despite many initiatives, e.g. National Association of Health Authorities (1988), to enhance the understanding and quality of work experiences for black nurses, there is very little published work of their experiences, and little evidence that these experiences have improved since the work of Lee-Cunin (1989).

For the purpose of this chapter, the term 'black' will be used to include all non-white ethnic minorities. The aim here is to highlight the nature of the contemporary black nurses' experiences.

It is desirable that every assertion or statement made is substantiated by research work carried out empirically. The credibility of a piece of work is highly regarded if the statements and assertions have empirical and statistical significance. However, the fact that there is not much work carried out in this area makes such an exercise impossible. The more poignant point here is to ascertain why, despite so many cases of discrimination at workplaces being heard at Industrial Tribunals (CRE 1997), there is so little published work about the plight of black nurses.

It is generally accepted by the academic world that the merit of good scholarly work is marked by robust research, with a large random sample and a powerful methodology with an equally potent statistical significance. However, while this notion is not disputed, its heuristic value is questioned for the purpose of citing awareness of the plight of black nurses and their experiences. What would it actually mean to quote studies that may state that the experiences of black nurses are positive and they are euthusiastic about their practices; or the antithesis, that the black nurses' experiences are ones of prejudices and unfairness? If one accepts the former statement emanating from empirical studies, that the experiences of black nurses are positive, then that would not be re-flecting the experiences of contemporary black practitioners. On the other hand, if the empirical studies were to say that the experiences of black nurses are bad and unfair, then we could argue that the reasons for such outcomes could be attributed to bad sampling, biased interpretation, poor analysis and so on. Such evaluation would negate the findings and value of previous studies and may not offer any more information in ascertaining or understanding the current experiences of black practitioners.

However, studies that have specifically focused on black staff experiences, i.e. Lee-Cunin (1989), Beishon, Virdee and Hazell (1995) and anecdotal cases collected for this study, have highlighted widespread adverse experiences by black practitioners.

What this tells us is that whatever inquiries, plans and policies that have been created and implemented to bring about justice for black ethnic minorities are not filtering through to practice areas. Similar inference is also made by Beishon *et al.* (1995). It further leads to the assertion that all the above initiatives were no more than paper exercises, because if they were anything more then these anti-discriminatory practices and equal opportunity policies would have ensured that not a single contemporary black nurse would have felt the pain of unfair treatment, prejudicial remarks and appalling working conditions and treatment. At the very least, improvements would have been evident. The obvious question then is why these initiatives have not had the desired impact in bringing about a better quality of work experience for ethnic minorities?

Why have the NHS leaders and managers not reacted to the adverse experiences of black nurses? Several explanations may exist, but the most frequently articulated relate to the managers themselves not appreciating the extent of these traumatic experiences. In some cases this is because they are truly not aware of the sentiments and adverse experiences, but on other occasions it is because they are indifferent. There are some managers and leaders who are indifferent because they don't care; while others may truly care but give the impression of indifference because they do not have the understanding and measures to deal with these rather sensitive issues.

In other instances, there is the perception amongst some employers that, given the NHS is one of the largest employers of black nurses, then the NHS must be offering equality of opportunities. However, this is far from being the case, and nurse leaders and managers must be fully cognizant of the problems black nurses experience and must make efforts to ensure the organisations and work environments are free of prejudicial attitudes and behaviours.

THE REALITY OF EXPERIENCE

The experience of being different was well articulated by Mary Seacole (1857), when she remarked, 'they shrank from accepting my help because it flowed from a somewhat duskier skin than theirs' (cited in Alexander *et al.* 1984).

So what has happened over the last one hundred and forty years in relation to ensuring that carers from diverse backgrounds are equally valued and cared for by employers? The answer appears to be very little (Beishon *et al.* 1995; Wing 1991). It is ironic that despite so many advances in so many areas of human living, medicine and technology, there is little improvement in ensuring that ethnic minorities receive equality of opportunity and experience in the nursing profession. Black nurses, like all nurses, want to offer care to those in need. They wish for no more than humanity, fairness and equal opportunities to be offered by the employers; fair treatment and an environment free of racial harassment from the colleagues they work with and the clients they care for. Is this really so much to ask?

Feelings are aroused when unfairness prevails because of ethnicity. However, there is a need to express caution, for it is not the case that all black nurses are treated adversely or experience hostile encounters. Nor is it the case that all black nurses themselves are without prejudice and all that they do is just and humane. No, as with any ethnic group forming a proportion of a professional group, one will find a number who are less competent, less committed, or motivated by other than professional values.

However, this chapter is not going to concentrate on the necessity for punitive measures for this group, as there are many in existence. What this chapter wishes to concentrate on is the black nurse who works hard, who delivers good care, who is highly professional, but who goes unnoticed and disadvantaged in various aspects of professional development and work experience.

One has only to look at the nursing literature to note how frequently Florence Nightingale is mentioned, quoted, praised and highly regarded. But what of Mary Seacole, who served in Crimea with Florence Nightingale, whose humanitarian and medical services to the British army in the period of 1854 to 1856 led to her receiving deserved recognition from individual soldiers and also from Queen Victoria? How many nurses have heard of this lady or know of her contributions? Decades later: 'there is little mention of this black nurse' (Lee-Cunin 1989); 'but with less fame' (Wing 1991). After one hundred and forty years, such unfairness still prevails, such injustice still exists.

Much of the content for this chapter is based on observations of practices in the clinical environment in varied hospital settings over a period of four years and includes many anecdotal accounts of overt racial discrimination in current hospitals. Most of these examples refer to black nurses' experiences in psychiatric settings, but there is no doubt that black nurses in other specialities encounter similar experiences. As one reads this chapter, there will be many other black nurses experiencing unjust treatment in some form of professional development, or harassment in the work environment.

The chapter will further examine why such unfairness prevails and will examine relevant policies and measures which have been put in place to counter such inequalities in the workplace. Questions will be raised as to why some black nurses experience unfair treatment and others do not. What really is the difference that leads one group of black nurses to be successful and another to fail? Is it really all the fault of the NHS or the white nurses, or can any of the adverse experiences of black nurses be attributed to themselves, in some cases perhaps inadvertently, and if so how? An explanation will be offered with recommendations to eradicate the real and perceived adverse experiences of black nurses.

So what is the evidence? How widespread are these adverse experiences felt by black nurses? Beishon et al.'s (1995) study estimated that eight per cent of NHS staff are from ethnic minorities and the study identified disparity between equal opportunity policies on the one hand and actual practices in the workplace on the other. Data obtained from six nurse employers, one hundred and fifty interviews and a postal survey of more than fourteen thousand staff revealed that many nurses felt that the allocation of training and promotion opportunities were unfair. Racial harassment of ethnic minority staff by patients and colleagues was widespread. Nurses and midwives did not think that management was doing enough to tackle the problem of racial harassment. Ethnic minority nurses, in particular black nurses, had not advanced as far along the grading structure as their white colleagues, even after controlling for other career factors such as qualifications and length of time in the profession. Similar comments were received from many contemporary practitioners, and unfairness in promotions were witnessed in the clinical settings.

Agbolegbe's (1984) study of six health authorities in the south of England was one of the most revealing of racial discrimination within the NHS. Concerned about the findings, Agbolube suggested the need for a systematic study of the experiences of ethnic minority nurses in the NHS and a comprehensive examination of the attitudes of health authorities towards equal opportunities. In addition, the need for a nationally agreed monitoring device to ensure equitable representation of ethnic minority nurses at all levels was also sought. However, thus far there has been a poor response and little effort has been made to ensure these measures are activated.

Hick (1982) noted that the main role of ethnic minority nurses was one of subservience and low status within the profession. Lee-Cunin (1989) stated: 'Most nurses reported, irrespective of the qualifications of black nurses, that many could only pursue SEN courses and widespread unfair promotional opportunities were evident.'

The London Association of Community Relations Councils (London Association of Community Relations Councils 1988) found overwhelming evidence of lack of equal opportunities in the employment practices of London Health Authorities. They further added:

> the overall performance of Health Authorities in London in tackling racial disadvantage and discrimination in employment is deplorably poor ... fifteen months after the introduction of the CRE code of practice and seven years after receiving the clear policy advice of DHSS, Circular HL (78) 36, most of them have achieved very little and some have attempted nothing.

The LACRC confirms the general evidence from the literature, and the anecdotal accounts, of widespread lack of opportunities for personal and professional development for contemporary ethnic minority nurses within the NHS.

Beishon et al. (1995) urged the need for procedures for recruitment and promotion to be concise, and the people involved to be trained in their use. She also recommended that special attention be given to those who have been discriminated against in the past.

Beishon et al.'s (1995) study found, in both their qualitative interviews and the quantitative survey, widespread and often blatant racism within working relationships and racial harassment from patients. Management was not seen to be doing anything. Their statistical analysis made the first step in suggesting that black nurses were disadvantaged in an array of professional development and promotion opportunities. Findings from Akinsanya (1988) indicated widespread discrimination in training opportunities, promotions and in clinical settings from both patients and peers.

Lee-Cunin's (1989) anecdotal account of black nurses' experiences also found under-representation of black nurses in senior and management positions.

In Protasia Torkington's (1987) study of two hundred nurses, 33 per cent of black nurses had to wait for periods of two to six years for promotion, while only 1.2 per cent of white nurses had to wait the same period. Lee-Cunin (1989) also found black nurses were treated unfairly when they sought promotion.

When they did succeed in gaining promotion they were subjected to so much unjust process that often their performances were affected, and most relinquished their position – thus reinforcing the view that black nurses could not cope.

RACISM FROM PATIENTS

What happens when a patient levels racial remarks? It has often been the case that when patients have levelled racial remarks overtly, black nurses have often had to be tolerant as these remarks were made by 'patients' – i.e. they are ill, therefore pay no heed to them, or in other cases because they are mentally ill. Discrimination is also experienced by black nurses in clinical and domestic settings whilst in the process of delivering care. Usually these black nurses, though disturbed and perturbed by these remarks, continue to engage in their caring and nursing duties. There are, however, questions that need to be raised. Were the remarks made because of mental illness, or were the remarks made because of personal dislike, i.e. because the nurse was of a different origin? The question really is, should the black nurse continue to tolerate such inflammatory remarks. Can racism of any nature, from any person, ever be justified? After one hundred and forty-one years, since the first recorded remark of 'colour' in Alexander's text (1984), in our society of multi-ethnicity, where equal opportunities and treatment are said to be the norm, it is not justified to continue to tolerate and condone such activity.

In the case of consumers, they have to be discouraged from continuing such prejudicial behaviours by the nursing practitioners, by colleagues, by the families, by the hospital and its management. In cases where racism prevails, the black practitioner must have the right to refuse to care for the discriminatory patient. This needs to be carried out in a professional manner: first the nurse's concerns should be brought to the attention of the patient; if these efforts fail, then the nurse must bring this to the attention of the senior nurse, and hopefully such an intervention will stop the unacceptable behaviour. If it continues then future care for the client will be offered by a different nurse, as long as the client's well-being will not be affected in any way by the change to a new practitioner. In extreme circumstances, the authorities may implement more stringent policies, to the extent that patients holding such racially discriminatory views will not be cared for by the establishment.

If the reasons are explored as to why, after all these years, racial taunts and overt discrimination continue, then there emerges a helplessness phenomenon experienced by black practitioners, like that identified by Lee-Cunin's (1989) study. It is as though the black practitioner has been conditioned to expect such unfavourable treatment, so that they ignore the abuse, tell the patient not to be abusive, or walk away. When the abuse takes place other patients may laugh and, although it is difficult to appreciate, other staff members may also engage in the humour, to the extent that the offended black practitioner leaves the clinical environment. Nothing more may happen and the affected practitioner is left uncertain and demoralised. Telling the patient off could result in a reprimand by senior nursing colleagues, or lead to disciplinary action. Communicating feelings of unease and disquiet to colleagues may lead to responses which trivialise and devalue the nurse's experience.

Over the years, such situations have been experienced, but they must stop. They can be stopped, and this can be achieved collectively. Hospitals have robust overt anti-smoking policies which have taken no more than fifteen years to become a force. So, why can't there be similarly effective anti-discriminative policies? Some would argue that there are already such anti-discriminative policies, such as the initiative of NAHA (1988), therefore the problem is not one of having policies but rather the effective means of implementing them.

As was evident in Beishon et al.'s (1995) study, the policies were not filtering through to the workplaces, and measures necessary to ensure equality were never evident. So what needs to be done is to ensure that clear and practical measures are accessible and operational in all clinical environments and all practitioners informed of these measures. This can be done, perhaps not overnight, but at least it can be set in motion. The issue must be addressed jointly by patients, nurses and the establishments, to ensure that no single person has to experience pain on the basis of their different ethnicity when all they want to do is to care for those in need. Racial remarks and behaviour by nurses towards ethnic minorities must become a disciplinary matter. Unless clear and enforceable measures are in place, no change will occur.

Education policies, guidelines and information brochures must all carry an active anti-discriminatory message. Nursing colleagues of all backgrounds must assist to ensure that the abuse is eradicated. They must begin to create an environment less traumatic and inflammatory, and fairer for the next generation. If these measures are not engaged in now, then the abuses will continue. The clinical settings must change. Black nurses must stop being helpless – they need to be strong and accept nothing less than a non-discriminatory environment.

FAILURE TO CHANGE THE CULTURE

A decade since Lee-Cunin's (1989) study and the initiative of NAHA (1988), what is different? Sad to say, nothing much. In the author's recent clinical experience many problems and difficulties continued to be experienced by black nurses.

In one clinical environment where the author was a practitioner many unsatisfactory experiences and practices were witnessed. Black nurses became discouraged from applying for promotion as, after several attempts, they reached the conclusion that they would not get the post. They also freely stated that they believed the reason why they would not get a post was not because of their lack of ability but because they were black.

It was very disturbing to notice excellent carers in such helpless positions. They were unable to do much – there was no one to turn to, to fight their case. Feelings of anger and disillusionment were widespread. Non-black staff could be promoted after only three months with fewer qualifications and less experience. There were occasions where senior posts were never externally advertised and had only one applicant. No black nurses applied because word had already gone round that the post was already occupied and the appointment was a mere formality. On one occasion, a nurse was appointed to an F Grade post while still under investigation for professional misconduct. She was the only applicant and was perceived by staff to be 'well connected' to the hierarchy of the establishment. The practitioner had only been in post for a relatively short time, and had very little experience and had no leadership skills, no knowledge of the speciality and often had been the stimulus for aggressive incidents.

There were also reports of blatant initiatives by senior nurses to appoint and promise senior grades on the basis of being their 'right-hand man'. Such promises meant that instructions given by the senior nurse must be followed.

On one occasion, such an initiative brought about an adverse experience for a black senior enrolled nurse. He was perceived not to be 'up to it', therefore he was subjected to a number of tasks in which sometimes the expectations were unrealistic and dangerous – for example, admitting a patient in a secure unit without any assistance. On this occasion there were nine staff on duty, and when colleagues offered to assist with the admission, they were warned off by the ward manager's 'right hand man'. When they, concerned and dismayed with such measures, brought their concerns to the ward manager, he stated that these measures were necessary in order to ascertain the nurse's competence.

The ward manager was asked if he had seen the nurse in question and discussed with him the areas of concern in professional practice, and if further training and development was provided and a period of time given to facilitate progress in the areas of practice of concern. No such measures were ever in place. This clearly was not an exercise to enhance the nurse's practice, but measures more likely to dissuade the practitioner from continuing to be an employee. Such punitive measures should have no place in any nursing environment and no practitioners of any origin should be subjected to such bullying tactics. On this occasion they wanted him out, and they sadly did succeed in doing so, after subjecting him to a number of distressing situations. Yet in this very environment there were numerous non-black practitioners whose practice and professional standards were highly questionable. Needless to say the ward manager had been the only internal applicant for the post, and had been appointed without any internal or external competition.

The pivotal role in the clinical area is that of the ward manager. This post is vital to ensure that clinical excellence, staff development and good practices prevail. However, different ward managers interpret their roles and functions differently. There is often poor clinical leadership and role modelling, and many assume a more managerial role and less of a clinical role. The clinical environment is at present desperately in need of clinical leaders to lead good practice – yet the right person in this role could make a significant contribution to eradicating prejudices and discriminatory practice. Just imagine if the person occupying this role is indifferent about these issues, or advocates these views. The need for ward managers as such must be questioned – the clinical environment needs good clinical practitioners and leaders, not managers.

The work of Lee-Cunin (1989), Beishon *et al.* (1995) and Wing (1991) highlighted both racism and poor opportunities for black nurses to occupy senior positions. Black nurses face barriers at every stage of their careers. The reason why so few black nurses get promoted to senior positions is not because of lack of ability or experience, poor education or poor professional practice, but because they are black. Such sentiments were strongly articulated by the black nurses in Lee-Cunin's (1989) and Beishon *et al.*'s (1995) studies. Similar experiences continue to be expressed by black practitioners today. There are many black nurses, very well qualified, who do not get promoted.

Take the case of X, functioning as a staff nurse at E Grade for nineteen years in a psychiatric unit. During this period he had applied for an F Grade post eight times. Of the eight times, he was shortlisted three times, but never got the post. However, he had acted at the higher grade on five separate occasions, on one occasion for as long as eleven months. Most recently, the post he applied for was given to a white staff nurse of eleven months' experience and with lesser qualifications. Naturally, this led to the conclusion that X did not get the job because he was black. This black nurse stated that he would not apply for any more promotions. Other black nurses also said that a black nurse would not be promoted in this unit.

It could be argued that the white nurse got the post because he had done well in the interview and had innovative ideas for practice etc.; but often there is no follow-through to assist or explain to candidates why they fail to get the job. On other occasions, there have been few or no opportunities for a practitioner who failed to obtain promotion to be given support and help to enable him or her to succeed the next time.

In the absence of such measures, the conclusion is made that the practitioner failed because he/she was black. Black nurses are not asking for any favours; they don't want any special privileges. All they want is a system that gives equal opportunities to all, where promotions to senior positions are made on merit. Such a process has enormous desirability, for example in enhancing the quality of care, providing good promotional role models and good mentors for trainee nurses, and allowing feelings of justice and good morale to prevail in the working environment. There should consequently be fewer practitioners going off sick, better continuity of care, and more incentive for ethnic minorities to join the nursing profession.

Given such difficult circumstances, how are black nurses coping? Several different patterns appear to emerge. Some black staff choose to engage in academic studies to change their careers. They do so by funding themselves, leaving the NHS and becoming permanent agency nurses. By doing so, it enables them to earn more money but invariably compromises both their professional and family lives. Many work very long hours and have few days off. In some areas of the country, many of the night nurses are from the black community. Although this is a feature highlighted in Lee-Cunin's (1989) study, unlike her period of ten years ago where it was possible to have senior positions on nights, such opportunities are far less today, as many establishments have twenty-four-hour rotations in place. As such, opportunities for promotion are scarce. However, the number of black nurses on night duty remains high, and yet again this has become necessary to get away from injustice, undesirable policies and prejudices during the daytime. For many this has become the only way to earn more money, continue their studies and to work at a time in which there are likely to be minimal harassments. All at a cost to the black nurse and the establishment.

EFFECTING CHANGE

The initiatives of NAHA (1988) should by now have contributed to a more just and fair working environment. Yet the evidence from the floor is still one of unfairness and a perception that employers are indifferent, and active prejudicial notions continue to exist. It does increasingly appear that the need to improve opportunities is rather a complex one. Mere policies will not suffice. Beishon et al. (1995) concluded their study by highlighting the need for a relationship between policy and practice. They recommended that policies implemented to monitor equal opportunities and discrimination must also be evaluated for their effectiveness. They further urged the need to review the developmental and promotional prospects of individual nurses, especially black nurses near the band of E and F grades. Finally, they highlighted the need to campaign to make every employer and employee feel responsible for supporting ethnic groups and preventing racial harassment.

These parsimonious recommendations must filter through to all employers and employees. Covert prejudicial practices are still widespread today. Measures must be in place to eradicate these cancerous practices, which do great harm not only to black nurses but to the organisation as a whole.

Black nurses have a role to play too. There is no point in sitting back and hoping that one day things will change for the better. Hoping alone is not enough, nor is it sufficient to expect health authorities and statutory bodies and their policies to eradicate racism. These policies alone will not suffice, as evidence over the decade and recent anecdotal reports testify. Policies can only work with the active participation of all concerned.

However, there was something else that was very evident in the clinical environment described earlier. This was that the prejudicial experiences were shared amongst themselves and there was no effort on the part of the black nurse who experienced prejudicial treatment to squash the unjustness. Instead, he or she related the adverse experience to a fellow black nurse and the fellow black nurse who hitherto had not experienced any prejudicial experience became conscious of racial discrimination. One black nurse's adverse experiences sometimes prejudices the outlook of other black nurses, in that they will not apply for promotion in a place where a colleague has already failed because, they believe, he was black. Therefore black practitioners sometimes reason that the application will be a futile endeavour as they will also fail to get promoted because they are black. So the reason why the black nurse does not apply for promotion has nothing to do with the employers but with the black peer groups and the anticipated outcome.

The phenomenon of helplessness is sometimes perpetuated by black nurses themselves. Negative feelings and attitudes prevail from other peers' experiences. While it may be true that a black nurse did not get promoted because of his ethnicity, it does not follow that this would be the case for all black nurses. Black nurses must continue to act positively, encourage one another, help one another, continue to support all black colleagues. Black nurses must continue to apply, fight, challenge and question. There is no room for fear of adverse consequences. There are sufficient policies in place for one to activate to ensure unfairness does not prevail.

When a black nurse experiences prejudice choosing not to do anything about it only makes the working environment difficult for fellow colleagues. That is how unjust and unfair management systems are allowed to persist. If black nurses continue to be fearful, and differ, and not fight, generation after generation will continue to experience adverse experiences.

Some measures that may help the cause of equal opportunities are suggested below. Some are already required as part of employment law; others are practices which could serve to prevent or alleviate the situations defined in this chapter.

The recommendations are as follows:

1.   Appropriate equal opportunity policies and anti-discriminatory practices, with consequences for offenders, must be in place in all organisations.

2.   All policies must be clear and easily accessible.

3.   All organisations must have an equal opportunities adviser, with the power to eradicate adverse discriminatory practices.

4.   All applicants failing a promotion must be given feedback so that they recognise their deficiencies, and appropriate support and training must be provided to enable them to improve their observed weaknesses. The process must be sensitive, fair and supportive.

5.   All interview panels must have an equal opportunities adviser, either from within or outside the organisation.

6. Where a post is internally advertised, then the interview panel must have an external representative to prevent bias and to ensure a fair process.

7. For appointments to higher-level positions, an external prominent figure must be an inherent part of the interview panel.

8. Every organisation must establish a neutral body accessible to all practitioners for expressing their experiences of prejudice. Such a body will also help to correct any erroneous perceptions that may have been formed by a practitioner's promotion (or lack of it).

The care provided in hospitals generally reaches out to all in society, a society of many cultures and diverse ethnicity. In the interests of excellence, the care team must reflect the society it serves, and allow all to achieve their goals and objectives. Black nurses must be free of prejudicial experiences.

Much needs to change to bring about a humanitarian working environment without which client care will suffer, and the organisation itself at best will only provide a fragmented service. It is difficult to appreciate how a caring profession can be so dedicated to caring for so many, but not for those who serve side-by-side to achieve the caring.

CHAPTER 14

Black Women Patients in the Forensic Service

Margaret Orr

As part of the course entitled 'Working With Difference' run by Charles Kaye, Tony Lingiah and Chandra Ghosh in the Training and Education Centre at Broadmoor Hospital, I lead a seminar entitled Other Challenges of Providing Equitable Care for Black Women. I present four cases to illustrate some of the major issues. Clearly we cannot make broad generalisations from four cases, but their tragic stories are live examples of some of the problems raised by their colour, culture, gender, mental state, trauma, lack of support systems and society's attitude to their offending. This chapter raises more questions than answers and is deliberately provocative, hopefully to improve services. To help put their stories in context the ethnic grouping of the patients in Broadmoor Hospital in September 1998 is shown in Table 15.1.

All women who have been admitted to Broadmoor Hospital over the past five years have been deemed too dangerous to be treated in medium security. All are assessed on the same criteria for dangerousness as men (absconding risk, arson risk, use of weapons, targeting of victims, etc.) but there remains a suspicion that women are more likely than men to be admitted due to inadequate facilities for their needs in medium security (e.g. same sex wards), difficult or disruptive behaviour (e.g. repeated deliberate self harm) or because they require prolonged length of stay (most medium secure units still expect a maximum of 2 years although there are frequent exceptions). It is believed that black and white women are equally liable to this potential for escalation to high security admission, but there is a need for more in-depth analysis of referrals from prisons and medium secure units to clarify whether the same proportion of black as white women are referred and what is the true morbidity within the female prison population. There are fewer women than men in medium security and there are even fewer black women and it is possible that they are even more often referred to high security.

Table 14.1 Ethnic grouping of patients in Broadmoor Hospital, September 1998

Current Patients	Male	Female	Total
Not known	13	1	14
White	261	65	326
Black Caribbean	45	9	54
Black African	6	3	9
Black other	6	1	7
Indian	4	0	4
Bangladeshi	1	0	1
Chinese	1	0	1
Other ethnic group	9	1	10
Not given	1	0	1
Total	347	80	427

Common features of the four women described below are that they are all black, of African-Caribbean origin, and are second generation, i.e. born in England to black parents. They are all of child-bearing age and are, or were, all detained under hospital orders with restriction by the HO on discharge (Section 37/41 of the Mental Health Act 1983). All were of average intelligence or above and none were considered to have a personality disorder at the time of admission. Two remain in the hospital and two have been transferred to medium security.

Case study 1

Miss A was the first child born to a single parent who had come to the UK to join her childhood sweetheart, but the marriage ended at the time Miss A was born. Her mother, who worked as a cleaner, went on to have two further pregnancies with different men. The second daughter is believed to have been brought up by her father and the third pregnancy, when Miss A was 13 years old, ended in a male child who died within hours of birth at hospital. Miss A had attended normal school till then with no obvious problems. She developed a depressive illness with anger directed towards her mother. Miss A began to truant from school, and was regarded as out of parental control but refused to attend child guidance with her mother. She was arrested frequently by the police under Section 136 of the Mental Health Act 1983, was regarded as promiscuous, an alcohol abuser and repeatedly violent, but had no substantial hospital admissions. At 18 she committed the offence which brought her to Broadmoor Hospital by allegedly trying to attack a neighbour's child with a knife. She was unfit to plead and was sentenced under the Criminal Procedures Insanity Act (CPIA).

In Broadmoor Hospital she was violent, psychotic despite medication, with thought disorder, auditory hallucinations and multiple delusions relating to babies and staff. She was often comforted by staff bringing her sweets and chocolate. Obesity became a problem. She spent many hours in seclusion due to her level of disturbance.

Discussion points from this case study are:

1. There was a lack of support for Miss A's mother from social services, from health and from education. (What was offered and what could she accept? What was the understanding of the society in which she found herself abandoned without her own family? What support did the black society offer her?)

2. There was frequent use of Section 136 of the Mental Health Act 1983 (detention by police and taken to a place of safety) with inadequate follow-up by health services after police correctly identified the mental health need. (Has the Clunis report improved cases like this by improving health and local authority liaison? Is continuity of care even less for blacks than for whites? If so, why is this?)

3. Was there poor representation at time of trial? She was unable to give evidence. There were poor records of arrest available for future work and assessment of risk. (Is there enough support at time of trial for legally naïve defendants? What are the advocacy services like now for young black clients?)

4. Staff response was well meant but inappropriate for the patient's needs. (Do we have enough black staff in each discipline? If the staff are black but African and the patient is African-Caribbean does that help the patient? Who are her role models? Is this important?)

5. Now in hospital there is no appropriate advocate – she has exhausted supportive groups such as Women in Special Hospitals (WISH), Afro-Caribbean Mental Health Association (ACMHA) and League of Friends. (How can the black community be more involved in secure psychiatric services? How can we remove the stigma of mental disorder and of offending related to that disorder in the black as well as the white community? Are these issues more stigmatising in black society? Can the black churches be invited to contribute?)

Case study 2

Miss B was the middle child of a large intact family, where her father and mother were in regular employment and provided a good standard of living but little emotional warmth. She developed severe depression in her mid-teens and began abusing alcohol as well as making multiple attempts to commit suicide interspersed with using deliberate self harm to relieve emotional pain. There were frequent admissions to psychiatric hospital, some lengthy and associated with violence and attempts to set fires. After the longest period in the community supported by CPN, social worker, psychotherapist, ACMHA and day centre attendance, cutbacks in services resulted in anger and feelings of rejection with the setting of a serious fire and subsequent admission to Broadmoor Hospital in a depressive state with auditory hallucinations and paranoid delusions. In therapy she has revealed serious and prolonged childhood sexual abuse, but she is making steady progress.

Discussion points from this case study are:

1. There is a need to understand what underlies deliberate self harm and symptoms of borderline personality disorder and identify culturally significant methods of treatment and assessment.

2. There is a need to recognise and treat addiction to alcohol. Abuse of solvents and drugs in black women may go unrecognised.

3. How often do we consider a trauma basis, and in particular childhood sexual abuse, in the pathogenesis of mental disorder in the black population?

4. We must recognise that paranoid delusions may be symptoms of distress, not always from schizophrenia but as part of the reaction to society's racist attitudes.

5. Apparently small 'cutbacks' in service may seem to leave an adequate support network, e.g. the legal requirements of the Care Programme Approach (CPA) standards may be fulfilled, but the true needs of a patient may not be identified. Readmission may be necessary for some patients when frequency of community visits falls below a critical level. Community care needs the support of in-patient beds at time of crisis.

Case study 3

Miss C's family was intact and both parents worked to provide for their family, the rest of whom succeeded. By mid-teens Miss C was indulging in social drugs, alcohol and solvent abuse. She joined a pop group going as a 'follower' to the continent where she had a psychotic breakdown resulting in hospital admission and transfer to the UK. She had three illegitimate children by the age of 26 (her first at 17) and was supported by her parents although living separately. She had several hospital admissions for the treatment of schizophrenia but was living with her two younger children in her own house when she stabbed and injured her visiting consultant psychiatrist. She was not obviously psychotic but later revealed her feelings of insecurity and need for containment which had been present for six weeks since a burglary of her home. She responded to regular depot medication in Broadmoor Hospital and was able to transfer to medium security after some years.

Discussion points from this case study are:

1.   Assessment of risk in the community must consider the stress of what seems a troublesome but not life-threatening event to most of us but devastating to the person with mental illness or who is particularly vulnerable. Illegitimacy, for some African-Caribbean families, can be disastrous, alienating them from their church and support network.

2.   Drugs may precipitate schizophrenic illness but they have not been shown to cause it. There needs to be education on drugs and the part they play in illness in the black community as well as the white.

3.   Social pressures from families can be overwhelming. Attitudes to mental illness by the patient's parents and their friends can undermine therapy or support it.

4.   Support to this woman's parents needs to increase as they get older, not be eliminated or curtailed. She requires her own social worker in addition to her children's social worker to enable her own needs to be addressed. The parents wish to return to the Caribbean but cannot leave their sick daughter and the grandchildren. These feelings require to be acknowledged and worked through by the multidisciplinary teams involved.

Case study 4

Miss D was the youngest of three sisters. She showed absolutely no abnormality in school or college apart from being the shyest of her family, with few close friends. She joined a religious sect with her elder sister. Miss D started visiting the charismatic sect leader in his home every evening where she was treated as a daughter by him and his wife. She began to believe he could control her body and gave her messages in her mind. She killed his wife in the belief he was instructing her to do so and came to Broadmoor Hospital for treatment of her chronic paranoid schizophrenia. She responded dramatically to medication, becoming well, but still had difficulties with making friends and her delusional system remained intact, i.e. she still felt controlled by her victim's widower. Now in medium security she is compliant with treatment and developing new living skills but will always require close supervision.

Discussion points from this case study are:

1. The family of this patient needed support and work relating to the offence. Fear of admission to Broadmoor Hospital is probably worse for the black community in view of the sudden deaths of three black male patients. It is important to explain to families and friends the circumstances of these deaths, to allow visits before admission for families and to provide support during visits.

2. There is a need to teach social, living and community skills to increase confidence, self-esteem and responsibility. Treatment is not just medicines and psychotherapy. For all patients an understanding of the role of religious beliefs and cultural values is important.

3. Close liaison between supervising psychiatrists and social workers to monitor risk with a cultural/religious sensitivity and understanding of the patient's belief system is crucial.

KEY ISSUES

I would like to make six further points considering these cases and having listened to the debates ensuing from them:

1. The effect of racism and lack of culturally sensitive attitudes on black women who are mentally disordered and who exhibit dangerous or criminal behaviour is seen in Miss A's case study. Frequent Section 136 arrests did not achieve the treatment she needed. Exuberance, disinhibition and vitality are often regarded as 'cultural', 'bad', 'typical of blacks' and no one seriously considered it was just as culturally inappropriate for a black woman to take off all her clothes and run out into the street as it would have been for a white woman. She was mentally ill for many years before diagnosis. The symptoms and signs exhibited by Miss B related to her feelings of guilt and poor self-esteem resulting from her sexual abuse, in addition to her 'illness', yet it was all too easy to fob her off as a 'black with a chip on her shoulder' or 'paranoid black' as stated so often.

   Police, GPs, social workers, psychiatrists, teachers and psychologists must look beneath the skin to the person and the distress before diagnosing and categorising.

2. There is a paucity of personality disordered black patients in the special hospital system and the question arises as to whether this is due to there being a reluctance to offer psychological therapies, a fear of criticism or lack of appreciation of what are the norms for black

society's personality profiles. It seems unlikely that there are such low numbers of personality disordered black people in the population. We wonder if there is poor recording or inadequate recognition of symptoms of disordered personalities or is there an underlying reluctance on the part of black people to acknowledge they may need help from the mental health services for what their own society regards as 'bad' behaviour.

3.   There would appear to be a reluctance to recognise depression as an entity in black women patients. Misses B, C and D had signs of lowered mood (abuse of alcohol, anxiety, deliberate self harm by overdosing and other psychological signs of depression). The externally directed hostility which may be the result of inner depressions is more often interpreted as 'badness' not 'sadness', but when emotions are not allowed expression but suppressed, sometimes for years, they may not be controllable by the person and result in outwardly directed violence.

4.   The recognition of sexual abuse among the black community may be even more difficult to acknowledge than in white society. The repugnance to accept and acknowledge that it occurs in ethnic minority communities seems to be an even greater barrier to dealing with it than in the UK generally. The amount is unknown but those of us who work with black women in Broadmoor Hospital have little doubt the level in the black community is likely to be as high as in the white. We need to discuss this more openly and help black women victims have the support they need. Schools and colleges need to be able to recognise signs of abuse (after disturbed nights), truancy (to hide the bruises), irritability, sleepiness, tiredness, withdrawal, sudden explosive outbursts (from high levels of fear and anxiety), watchfulness, bravado and tearfulness (from fear). All may be signs of abuse at home.

5.   It is a frequently stated myth that patients have drug-induced or alcohol-related psychosis. Our experience is that those who are admitted to our hospital may have had episodes of psychosis precipitated by drugs or alcohol, but there is almost universally an underlying psychotic/schizophrenic process illness. Our patients have illness and illicit drug-taking makes them worse even if they have symptomatic relief for short periods. Alcohol may be used to conceal symptoms, as in Miss B's case study, for many years before the full extent of illness is revealed. We must be very careful before attributing symptoms to alcohol or drug abuse.

6.   Finally, there is the question of providing a multidisciplinary staffing with experience of a variety of cultures and races to understand the

needs of our women, to support the families who are so often isolated (such as Miss A's mother). Our patients have often brought stigma to their families by their behaviour and now their place of treatment. Where pride in the family has been high, as in cases of Misses B, C and D, the ostracism by the rest of their 'friends' can be serious and unbearable. The shame and anger they feel needs compassion and sensitivity. Our staff need to support without patronising and understand without criticising.

THE WAY FORWARD

And so, for the future, what have we to offer black women in hospital? My patients have told me what they would like.

First, on the practical side, they would like expert advice on make-up to cover the scars of deliberate self harm. They would like to learn how to prepare and cook traditional African-Caribbean and African dishes. When they go on rehabilitation trips they want to visit the street markets and shops dedicated to their food and clothes. They feel more comfortable with escorts of their own colour but would rather go out with a white nurse than not at all.

When we spoke of their feelings and attitudes to illness they said they wanted to know about their past – both that of their own family and that of their people – but one woman said that she had shown her brother the video of *Roots* and he became so angry that he stopped seeing all his white girlfriends. She said that we need to discuss the meaning of the past for her people today.

It is already not enough to show documentaries and expect confused, mentally disordered minds to assimilate what is real and what unreal. Reality testing for someone with schizophrenia is very important. Our staff need to be aware of the culture and able to relate objectively. Group work dedicated to cultural issues for staff and patients should be part of our treatment care planning and specific sessions during induction courses are already planned. Our training course on working with difference is a start. Our patients should be more involved in future but it will be a gradual process as so few have the confidence to come forward. Empowerment of black women patients is still more difficult than for white women, and that is difficult enough. It has to be culturally acceptable empowerment if it is to work at all.

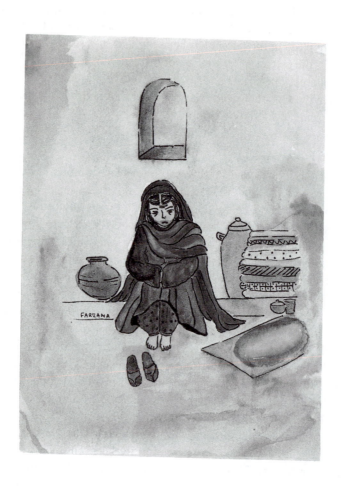

Depression – Farzona

CHAPTER 15

Asian Women
and Community Care

'Asian Khavateen'

Alia Khan

Poora jism dukhta hai. – Whole body is in pain. Dil pareshan hai – My heart
is worried. Sooch hi sooch me rehti hoo. – Always thinking, thinking.
(Tazeem, a Pakistani woman, member of ASRA)

This chapter is intended for those people whose work would bring them into
contact with women from the Indian subcontinent. I am a social worker from a
community mental health team in High Wycombe. Part of my workload involves managing a project called ASRA, a support group for Asian women with
mental health problems. The ASRA project was set up in 1992 by
Buckinghamshire County Council Social Services Department, and is staffed
by three workers, two of whom are Asian women volunteers. ASRA helps
women get in touch with themselves – they are encouraged to talk about their
lives in a safe environment in which they feel free to express their anger, fears
and tears in their first language, Punjabi. My role involves facilitating discussions and activities so that their participation encourages and develops their
identity, skills and abilities, necessary to empower their confidence in their various roles in the family and community. The content of this chapter includes experiences derived from women at ASRA. The women predominantly originate
from Azad Kashmir in Pakistan; a growing community in High Wycombe
which comprises 16 per cent of the local population.

This chapter seeks to complement the medical model of mental illness
which is predominantly used in treatment, because it is difficult to assist a person without an understanding of the social influences affecting them, both past
and present experiences. Tyler's (1874) definition of culture explains: 'that
complex whole which includes knowledge, belief, art, morals, law, custom, and

173

any other capabilities and habits acquired by man as a member of society'. Migration, *biradari* (kinship) and *izzat* (pride) also play a significant part in the personal and social development in Asian women. I shall be discussing these issues in both their cultural and social contexts, and shall conclude this chapter with some examples of the experiences of Asian women who have presented to existing mental health services and have found them inappropriate to their needs.

Unfamiliar behaviour and beliefs should be noted and understood in a social and cultural context, and should not be misinterpreted as mental illness. Culture is an important element of understanding why a person reacts badly to a certain situation and the response given by the society which is part of that person's secondary culture. Knowledge of immediate facts would assist the practitioner in the development of diagnostic tools which would be more relevant to the social and cultural context of Asian women in mental distress.

MIGRATION

To understand the social standing of women, it is important to direct your attention to the historical picture and the process of migration of the Asian population. The Indian subcontinent was under the rule of the British until 1948. At the time of independence the subcontinent was partitioned. States that were predominantly Muslim became Pakistan and those that were predominantly Hindu and Sikh became India and the migration across those borders caused a lot of pain and bloodshed. Differences between East and West Pakistan resulted in East Pakistan forming an independent country, called Bangladesh. Pakistan and India have an ongoing conflict to do with the claim to Kashmir.

Migration to Britain was encouraged by the British due to the postwar labour shortage. Smaller numbers of migrants came from areas around Rawalpindi and the North West frontier. In Azad Kashmir, the movement of the migrating population accelerated because of the political tension in Kashmir and by the forced evacuation of homes, as a result of the construction of the Mangla Dam. Urdu is the national language of Pakistan and is less spoken in the rural Kashmir region where schooling opportunities were limited. The smaller numbers who migrated from urban areas are generally literate in Urdu and English.

Since 1969 wives and children have had to establish their claim to an entry certificate by first obtaining 'entry clearance' from their British embassy or High Commission. This system was introduced to avoid delays at ports of entry to this country, by ensuring that dependents with a lawful right were checked before they left, and so-called 'bogus' applicants were weeded out. Total immigration from New Commonwealth and Pakistan has declined substantially, from 136,000 in 1961 and 1972 to 22,000 in 1988 (Skellington 1992).

At one time gynaecological examinations were common practice at Heathrow Airport and many women suffered the humiliation of unnecessary internal examinations. Many of these women were too old to enter Britain as dependants. There has been some progress towards stopping this degradation of Asian women – for example the British government brought pressure to bear to stop the virginity tests conducted abroad of immigrant women coming to Britain.

The use of X-rays to establish the age of potential immigrants has been condemned by the World Health Organisation. This practice is dangerous even when carried out by professional radiographers, but it is continually used in Dhaka, even on pregnant women, who under the Department of Health and Social Services regulations should only be X-rayed when medically essential. This practice has been carried out for years, but the people subjected to it have been too timid, apprehensive or vulnerable to expose the defects of the immigration system.

Even currently, Pakistani, Indian and Bangladeshi women wishing to join husbands and families in Britain experience endless interrogation, and can be excluded or sent to detention centres if Immigration is not fully satisfied by their intentions.

The Asian women coming to Britain for the first time, not knowing the language and uncertain of the future, are humiliated and degraded by the immigration system. This results in situations that, previously, the women could not have possibly imagined.

The effect migration has on Asian women is one of dislocation. Rack (1983) describes this to be a 'loss of role identity' and 'culture shock', a term first voiced by Oberg (1954).

> Parveen is a 52–year-old woman, diagnosed with depression, who always complains of physical pains. Psychosomatic symptoms are often coupled with a view that such patients do not understand that physical symptoms may be grounded in psychological stresses. Parveen expects treatment for the physical pain and does not connect the symptom to psychological stresses or does not relate to what is the basis of the pain.

This emotional state is precipitated when one's 'psychological cues', which may be the words, expressions and traditions that enable a person to function in a society, are replaced by new ones. Oberg also relates 'culture shock' to a form of mental illness, characterised by symptoms of trivial physical pains, paranoia, helplessness, refusing to learn the local language or meet with the host community and the pining to meet with one's own people. It could be argued that most Asians are protected from this state of despair as they choose to remain in a close-knit community and continue with the ways of life once lived in their homelands. Realistically, however, it is difficult to avoid life outside their community, and eventually a person will have to make contact with their doctor, local authority and others. Also, the life experienced within their communities does not fully reflect the life back home. For example, a woman who returns home from hospital after giving birth often visits her parents with her child for 6 weeks until she is well enough to return to her husband and continue with her role as a wife and assume the role of motherhood. This tradition cannot be practised in Britain if her parents live in Pakistan.

> Farah, aged 29, has suffered from postnatal depression since she gave birth to her son 5 years ago. She often pines for her parents and the feelings of togetherness once lived in Pakistan.

There has been research conducted under the auspices of the National Research Unit on ethnic relations which found that the majority of the Asian families in Britain are of the nuclear type. This has had a direct effect on Asian women, who, weakened by the separation from their families, suffering from the loss of mother, sisters and close friends, find themselves in a strange and unknown society. For many it is an especially distressing experience because the act of migration necessarily gives rise to social isolation. This together with the transfer of *biradari* (kinship) and *izzat* (pride) to the husband's family created a situation which is culturally irreversible in its effect. The concepts of *biradari* and *izzat* are explained as follows.

The identity of one's role gives a sense of security and recognition through socio-economic status, *biradari* and *izzat*. Security through employment, supported by credentials and skill, can be affected when an immigrant's qualification from back home may not be recognised in the Western world and may result in taking on a lower status of job role. Rack (1983) has mentioned that there is evidence to support that 'downward social mobility, in employment status terms, is a factor in the incidence of mental illness among immigrant groups'. However, role identity can also be influenced by patriarchal and matriarchal authority through the *biradari* system within the community.

Biradari (kinship)

Asian women come from many differing backgrounds. They speak different languages and practise different religious beliefs, the three main religions being Islam, Hinduism and Sikhism. Yet, apart from these differences they still share a majority of common experiences. Family life of these women follows an almost identical pattern. Life on the Indian subcontinent is reinforced through the joint family system. The joint family includes married brothers and unmarried sisters all living under the tutelage of the eldest male, which is usually the father or grandfather. Belongings are shared between the families and, if the family house is large enough, all members live within it. The head of the family has authority over all the others, and this includes those who are married or who are fathers themselves. The feeling of belonging to a group larger than just their immediate family is ingrained in people from rural India, Pakistan and Bangladesh. The migration process has not made a dramatic impact on the usual cultural values and migrations have generally been regarded as a means of enhancing their status and bettering their existing positions. The *biradari* or extended kinship group continues to have a major influence over individuals' activities and over their expectations of life in Britain. The *biradari* perpetuates itself through the institution of arranged marriages, which is crucial to its persistence and stability. Traditionally marriage is with first cousins and this has the effect of maintaining the *biradari* as kinship group.

Within the family the roles and functions of father and mother are well defined. The father is the provider and makes the decisions, while the mother's role is domestic and prescribed as such by both Islam and Hinduism. The family structure is based on patriarchal lines – the woman is not considered of any economic value even though she may work hard in the fields. Until she is married her success is not within her control. She is encouraged by religion, mythology and custom to produce sons. Her chief role therefore is as a producer of labour – her sons. If a woman has many daughters she is considered as unfortunate and a carrier of misfortune.

> Zubaida is a 50-year-old woman whose depression escalated when her husband married again because he blamed her for their childless marriage. She talks about lonely hours, sitting in her room, reminiscing vivid memories from her life before in Pakistan. She rarely leaves her home and only goes out when her transport arrives with a Pakistani female driver who escorts her to ASRA. She speaks no English and knows hardly anyone. Her isolation protects her from the fear of losing *izzat* (pride). This mountain of painful emotions is shared by many women.

Similarly, Rack (1982) suggests that loss of meaningful roles is one of the components of the syndrome of institutionalisation – the iatrogenic disorder that caused so many of the residents of the old-style mental hospital to sit all day sunk in apathy and inertia. 'What am I for?', if unanswered, leads easily to 'What am I?'

Izzat (pride)

For a woman, *sharam* – her shame and shyness is itself an honour. It can be described as a woman's pride because it reflects her purity and sensitiveness and is a common feature in all Indo-Pakistani cultures. The notion of *sharam* goes hand-in-hand with *izzat*. *Izzat* can be translated as honour and is a quality possessed by every individual, which can generally be negatively or positively affected by women, which then reflects the family as a whole:

> The sensitive and many faceted male family identity which can change as the situation demands it. From family pride to honour to self-respect and sometimes to pure male ego. (Wilson 1985, p.43)

The author also says that predictably it is women who place *izzat* most at risk. *Izzat* is a quality basic to the emotional life of Punjab. It is essentially male but it is women's lives and actions which affect it most. A woman can have *izzat* but it is not her own, it is her husband's or father's. Therefore, a woman's *izzat* is a reflection of the male pride of the family. A woman is encouraged to produce more males and if she fails society responds with oppression. Women in the peasant society were relied upon to reproduce the labour force so therefore the most important and uncontrollable facet in the peasant society occurred within a woman's body. This meant the woman's role made her the central symbol of the culture. She was the link between economic survival and the meaning of life.

The loss of identity also occurs when arranged marriages are renounced, which places the family's *izzat* at risk.

> Shazia is a 21-year-old who recently had an arranged marriage against her wishes. She attempted several suicides to escape the expectation of marriage imposed on her.

The study by Raleigh *et al.* (1990) analysed that between the ages of 15 and 24 suicide is a high risk factor for Asian women, who are 80 per cent more at risk than the general population. This percentage decreases with age. According to the 1971 Census, the 15–24-year-old age group is most at risk, 57 per cent being married and 47 per cent being single. The research was further discussed at a seminar conference, Asian Women and Suicide – Myths and Realities. Ravinder Radhhawa, author of two novels, *A Wicked Old Woman* and *Hari-Jan*, reminded us at the conference:

> life is about spirit with the actual body, longing for satisfaction with food, warmth and love, a magical spirit that can create music, dance, emotions but also distinguishes between right and wrong. Young women are subjected to hate, anger, violence and evil. This evil creates anger and despair which erodes all hopes and faith. To take away a person's hope is to kill their spirit. They feel life holds nothing for them. Suicide seems a way out – a last resort. We came to this country for a better life, we had our families, we started businesses. We were pioneers.

Wilson argues:

> Her role is at the heart, the core of civilisation. That is why she is kept in her place, if necessary by the most brutal oppression. If she rebels, the society itself may be overthrown. (Wilson 1985, p.9)

'To be kept in her place,' thought Nasreen, a 36-year-old woman with an unspecified mental illness. 'Me buri hoo buri – I am bad, bad. Muje safai ya kana pakana nahee hota – I don't do the cooking or cleaning. Buri hoo buri – bad, I'm bad. Vo muhje jooti se marhte he ... me buri hoo – he beats me with a slipper ... I'm bad.'

According to the 1992 British crime survey, 11 per cent of women who had lived with a partner had at some time experienced physical abuse (Mirrlees and Black 1995). Very little research has been done on Asian women and domestic violence, but a seminar event assisted by the West Midlands community focused on domestic violence in ethnic minority communities through an agency called WAITS. The analysis showed that there is an increasing number of reported incidents of domestic violence, up from 10, 350 in 1992 to 12,679 in 1994. Approximately 15 per cent of these involved members of the ethnic minority communities, in line with 14.6 per cent ethnic minority population in the area.

These Asian women's days are spent in loneliness and social isolation, cut off from family and social networks. They speak little or no English. Some are confined to their home, by their husbands or by their timidity, and they are seldom seen outside; others may become 'surgery haunters' – perhaps because a visit to the doctor is one of the few opportunities for a culturally-sanctioned outing (Rack 1990, p.290).

TREATMENT AND RESOURCES

Johannes Fassil (1996) undertook a national survey seeking the consumer perspective on primary health care for black and ethnic minority people. The analysis of the report found that GPs do not allow patients adequate time to explain their problems and symptoms. Furthermore, GPs do not take time to explain the treatment being suggested. This is particularly the case for non-English speaking patients. The reluctance of Asians to talk openly about mental health problems, or language and communication difficulties, may make it harder for GPs to recognise such problems should they arise.

The Commission for Racial Equality expressed concerns about primary healthcare in their position paper *The Race Implications of the Mental Health (Patients in the Community) Bill* (1995b). They noted that the standards of mental healthcare for Asian women are often not those offered to their white counterparts. The research also showed that ethnic minority people are more likely to be diagnosed as mentally ill and to have non-consensual powers used against them. Furthermore, the standard of care provision for ethnic minorities discharged from hospitals is often very poor.

The stigmatisation of mental disorder includes shame as well as fear. In Pakistan people only go to a psychiatrist if they are *paagal* – mad (in Britain this would equate to extreme psychosis). A person with other mental health problems is perceived as not *paagal*. Mental hospitals in Pakistan are rather nightmarish, where the common treatment is ECT. Staff are often uncaring and maybe cruel, few patients are ever discharged and all are compulsorily detained. If it became known that there was a 'streak of insanity' in a family it would affect the respectability not just of the individual but also of the whole family. This would seriously affect marriage prospects in a culture where marriages are arranged by elders. This stigmatisation may make the family prefer 'concealment to treatment' (Rack 1982).

> Razia, a former member of ASRA wept at one group meeting when she recounted her feelings of humiliation and betrayal because an interpreter had said to her, 'you need to see a doctor for mad people' in front of her in-laws. She was overcome by tears of shame and loss of *izzat*.

This resulted because of the lack of understanding and training of the interpreter and the weight of stigma, both covered with a layer of *izzat*. Culture and religion also play an important role in the need for Asian women to be seen by female workers. Asian women with limited English encounter problems with impartiality and confidentiality. If there is a small community who speak Punjabi, it can often be assumed that they all know each other. Similarly Rack (1982) states that 'even if there are, say, a thousand Bengali speakers in a city of half a million, it may be that those thousand form an enclosed community like a village within the city, and villages are notorious for gossip'. Women may therefore prefer not to be seen by a Punjabi speaker unless they are from a distant community.

CONCLUSION

There are concerns that there may be considerable unmet need for psychological support among black and ethnic minority populations, and that they may not be getting the right type of service they require. It has been found for example that Asian patients are often discharged into the community under the assumption that they will be looked after by 'the extended family'. This assumption is misguided, and has resulted in Asian patients being looked after by unqualified domestic carers, who are often isolated, with little practice, help or support.

Communication problems have been identified as a major problem in the diagnosis and treatment of illness in members of minority ethnic groups. The Commission for Racial Equality state that evidence has been found of a need for interpreters in mental health services, particularly for Asian patients. This provision is only partly met and is often largely supplemented by family members. Within communities this practice is widespread and writers including Richie (1964) have recommended it, but in practice Rack (1982) advises that it is unethical, unprofessional, uncivilised and totally unacceptable.

The Commission For Racial Equality Study (1989a) *The Experience of Health and Mental Health in an Ethnic Minority Group* indicated that GPs can be expected to continue to be the first and foremost point of service provision for Asian women with a mental health problem. GPs should therefore be in a position to have a good general knowledge and familiarity with the patients and their circumstances. However, there are aspects of primary healthcare services which may be considered as weaknesses. Among many practitioners there may be little understanding of aspects of Asian women's culture and social disadvantage. The study also recommends improvement to most primary care services with respect to mental health care.

The development of policies and services to meet the needs of Asian women requires innovations within and outside social services and the health service. Such innovation can include advocacy schemes and link-workers attached to GP consultation, other services in language provision, specialist workers in community mental health teams, including a bilingual psychiatric nurse and social worker; all of which provide a point of referral for GPs.

Discussed earlier were the life problems of Asian women which can be seen as mental illness but may require help by a non-medical service. The data from the CRE (1989a) study along with the experiences of the women from ASRA indicate some of the social, welfare and advice services needed, and which play a significant part in the alleviation of circumstances which cause mental distress. These support services include support for women with young children, housing advice and assistance, help after racial abuse and support from voluntary groups, and can play a considerable part in alleviating isolation and enhancing the capacity to cope.

I have tried to show how the female Asian community may often have specific needs which can affect their presentation and mental health. I believe it is therefore crucial for the services we provide to be appropriate to those needs and this necessitates involved professionals understanding the cultural issues and being sensitive and responsive to them.

PART IV

Effecting Change

CHAPTER 16

Making Policy Work

Jayne Hayes

INTRODUCTION

This chapter describes one medium secure unit's practical approach to developing services for patients from an ethnic minority background. It begins with statistical and geographical data about the Unit. The chapter continues by describing the impetus for improving services for these groups and how that change was planned. It then considers the implementation of that change through the use, mainly, of audit and training. The chapter concludes by setting out ongoing aims for the development of services for this group.

INTRODUCTION TO THE UNIT

This 27-bed Unit serves the needs of the mentally disordered offender population of Avon, Gloucestershire and Somerset. There are 12 acute beds with the added facility of an Intensive Care Area and 15 rehabilitation beds. Patients stay at the Unit for up to two years. There are two community psychiatric nurses attached to the Unit, carrying case-loads of patients discharged from the Unit. The Unit is funded for approximately 75 permanent professional staff, over 60 of whom are nurses. The Unit serves a predominantly rural area with two main conurbations – Bristol and Gloucester. In the South West of England (i.e. from Gloucestershire to Cornwall), 2 per cent of the population are from various ethnic minorities. It is likely that Bristol and Gloucester have the most significant ethnic minority populations in this region (Office for National Statistics 1997b).

At any one time 33 per cent of the in-patient population of the Unit can come from the ethnic minority groups. A snapshot of the patient group in 1997 revealed that the proportion of those from an ethnic minority, within or attached to the Unit, reduced as levels of security lowered. Whilst 36 per cent of the patients on the admission ward were from an ethnic minority, only 2 per cent of the community case load were. Six per cent of staff are from various ethnic minorities.

THE IMPETUS FOR CHANGE

A number of local and national issues led to the recognition that services for mentally disordered offenders from ethnic minorities needed to be developed at the Unit. National issues included the fact that the 1991 census found that 6 per cent of the British population were from ethnic minorities. It was clear that the over-representation of patients from an ethnic minority was not just an issue for the medium secure unit described. Yates and Craddock (1998) describe a medium secure unit where 62 per cent of the patient group were from the African-Caribbean community. Local issues included the Mental Health Act Commission visit reports (April 1997, October 1997) which noted that patients' case notes did not record patients' ethnicity and that staff were not aware of the need and purpose of ethnic monitoring. The Commission were also concerned that a patient had complained about racial abuse from a nurse. The complaint was fully investigated and was unproven. However, it highlighted that there were no harassment policies in the Trust and this led to some of the developments described later in this chapter.

Other things which led to the decision to develop these services were the fact that the senior nurse attended the course 'Working With Difference' at Broadmoor Hospital in the autumn of 1997 following her own interest in this area. There was also a concern in the Unit that the proportion of ethnic minority patients being referred to the Unit was increasing and that services provided for these patients felt unsatisfactory. The Mental Health Act Commission (1997) in their *Seventh Biennial Report* point out that provision across mental health services for patients from ethnic minorities is often 'basic and piecemeal'.

A number of different studies and reports (Fernando 1998; Department of Health and Home Office 1993; Prins *et al.* 1993) emphasise that there are inequities amongst ethnic groups in diagnosis, management, treatment and outcome. The impact of these inequities have been discussed earlier in this book by Inyama (Chapter 8) and Grant (Chapter 11).

PLANNING FOR CHANGE

The overall aim was to promote awareness and fairness in the care and treatment of those from an ethnic minority. This led to the development of policy strategy with the aim of providing the best service possible to all clients. Fernando (1998) argues that if forensic services can address and improve awareness of race and culture issues, this might 'be the key to improving services all round – for everyone.'

There is tremendous social, economic and cultural diversity between ethnic minority populations. Any strategy that attempts to develop services must avoid generalisation and stereotyping. This issue of stereotyping can be particularly problematic for psychiatry. Lewis, Croft-Jeffreys and David (1990) surveyed 220 psychiatrists using a case vignette. They found that varying the race and sex of the patient described in the vignette meant that the psychiatrists surveyed changed their clinical predictions. In particular these researchers were able to identify a stereotype of a black mentally ill person in the replies. The stereotype suggested that their illness would be of short duration and may involve aggression. Use of the criminal justice system was also considered more often than in the control group.

It is recognised that social economic deprivation and poor quality housing, often found in inner city areas such as those of Gloucester and Bristol, can lead to adverse effects on mental health and can significantly impact on those from ethnic minorities.

The experience of racism is a significant life event. It can occur in the NHS, the criminal justice system and society at large. McGee (1992) argues that racism is an issue that needs 'urgent and sustained action if the quality of health-care services to ethnic minorities is to be improved' (p.4).

The literature review and local knowledge was used to develop an action plan. Recommendations were made under the following headings:

1.   Clinical Development

2.   Recruitment and Training Developments

3.   Policy Developments

4.   Ongoing Developments.

MHAC (1997) and the Department of Health and Home Office (1993) give a checklist for the development of services for those from an ethnic minority. This includes consideration of appropriate physical care, staff training, the development of relevant policies and the involvement of advocacy groups. This information was used to help plan the local strategy which contained the following principal elements:

Clinical development

1.   The assessment documentation was reviewed, ensuring that cultural issues were taken into account.

2.   Racial harassment was recognised as a life event and included on all assessment tools.

Recruitment and training Developments

1.   Staff, at all levels, were to undergo cultural awareness training. Senior staff were to be encouraged to take the 'Working With Difference' course at Broadmoor Hospital.

2.   It was considered whether to advertise specifically for members of staff from the ethnic minority groups, taking into account that we currently have an ethnic minority staff population of approximately 6 per cent. Regular data was requested from the Trust Personnel Service.

3.   Every recruitment interview undertaken includes a question related to caring for ethnic minority patients. Some startling lack of knowledge has been shown by this simple change. In recent interviews for a senior nursing post the majority of candidates were unable to give any reasons why there was a higher proportion of patients from an ethnic minority within the Unit than that to be found in Britain in general.

Policy developments

1.   The Harassment Policy for racial and sexual abuse is clearly displayed in all clinical areas and implemented at all times. Patients or staff implementing this policy are offered managerial support to do so. All staff are educated about the impact of racism on individuals and trained in the use of this policy.

2.   There is effective statistical monitoring, as required by the Mental Health Act Commission, of those from ethnic minorities placed at the Unit.

3.   The relevant policies are reviewed annually, as part of the Unit's ongoing policy review system.

Ongoing developments

1.   A ward manager, through the appraisal system, was given responsibility for continuing to develop services for this area.

2.   Services for this group are regularly audited, the initial focus being to ensure the provision of appropriate food and physical healthcare.

IMPLEMENTING THE CHANGE

This section describes the 'how' of making the above changes.

New policy

The Harassment (Racial/Sexual Equality) Policy was written in May 1997, following a patient complaint, and is clearly displayed in all areas of the Clinic. Local social services harassment policies were used to inform its development. It is for both staff and patients.

The policy defines harassment as being:

Any behaviour which abuses, intimidates, humiliates, ridicules and/or undermines the confidence of a person or group due to their colour, nationality, ethnic group, disability, religious or sexual orientation or gender.

This definition is followed by a procedure for implementing the policy. The introduction of this policy was the first part of the process of developing services for those from an ethnic minority and raised staff and patients' awareness of relevant issues.

Training

The second step to implement the strategy was the development of a Cultural Awareness Training Pack used with staff. This evolved as a two-day workshop run by two senior nurses. The workshop gave information about cultural groups and allowed time to address attitudes and stereotypical beliefs. It included consideration of the individual attendee's own culture and facts, figures and research about the over-representation of black patients within the medium secure environment. It also included definitions of culture, ethnicity, race and racism and considered discrimination and anti-racist measures and the use of appropriate language. Black voluntary groups from the community were used to bring a richness and diversity to the teaching on the two days.

The discussions generated in the workshop about racism are of particular importance. As McGee (1992) points out, it is not possible to consider racism only intellectually. Any discussion about racism inevitably impacts on beliefs and attitudes. This was felt to be the most important aspect of the two days.

Fernando *et al.* (1998) argue that, as forensic psychiatry has a social control function, it is very important to ensure that racist perceptions do not influence judgements made. This makes it essential to give staff working in forensic areas anti-racist training and to implement anti-racist policies.

Attendees at the workshop are asked to 'action plan' to improve how their service cares for those from ethnic minorities. This programme has been run twice and is planned to run twice a year.

This is a similar training strategy to that described by Yates and Craddock (1998). They also describe a process whereby course attenders on a Cultural Awareness workshop were asked to 'action plan' to improve services for those from an African-Caribbean community.

Audit

The third action to implement the strategy was the audit. The audit was undertaken following the first set of Cultural Awareness Days in March 1998. The audit was designed to elicit the training needs of staff and to ascertain whether information on the specific needs of ethnic minority patients was available. The audit:

- established the number of patients in the Unit with specific cultural needs
- identified the religious and cultural needs of the patients, especially relating to personal care and dietary requirements
- ascertained whether these needs were being met
- provided a baseline for future audits and for developing standards of care
- identified areas in which staff required further training.

One questionnaire was given to all patients from ethnic minority groups, identified through the use of medical notes. The questions covered the patients' personal care, religious and dietary needs. Another questionnaire was distributed to all permanent nursing staff on both the acute and rehabilitation wards of the Unit. This was designed to identify the training needs of the nurses and to ascertain their knowledge regarding the personal care and religious and dietary needs of patients from ethnic minorities.

Eight patients from ethnic minorities were identified. Arrangements were made for the patients to be supported by staff in completing the questionnaire, if necessary. The patients were given a covering letter to explain both this arrangement and the purpose of the audit.

The outcome of the audit is presented here in two sections: the results from the patient questionnaire and the results from the staff questionnaire.

Patients

The sample of eight was obviously small. It did, however, represent the total number of patients from ethnic minority groups on the ward at the time of the audit. This represented approximately one-third of the in-patients on the Unit. The audit found that the majority of patients were satisfied that their religious and cultural needs were being met. One patient felt that staff were not sensitive to religious needs but made no further comment. Questionnaires of this sort are clearly problematic, particularly in relation to this sensitive area.

The patients may have felt that answering them honestly would affect care adversely and therefore may not have given true responses. However, the fact that there were only four questions and that they focussed on practical considerations may have limited this possible effect. The questions were:

1. Do your cultural or spiritual needs require you to use any special products for your personal care – e.g. hair, skin or beauty products?
2. Are you able to observe your religious beliefs?
3. Do you feel staff have been sensitive to your religious beliefs?
4. Do you require a special diet because of your cultural or religious beliefs?

The patients had to tick a box – 'yes' or 'no'. Room was given for comments but none were made. The purpose of the questionnaire was well explained – each patient received a covering letter and was offered extra support in its completion, if they needed it, from designated nursing staff. Patients were reassured, in the covering letter, that they would not be identified in any way. The simplicity of the questionnaire and the thorough explanation given were an attempt to get a true response from the patients. The level of reassurances given may have led to the patients becoming more suspicious rather than less about the purpose of the audit. An independent black advocacy group will probably be asked to assist in auditing the patients about these issues in the future. This may feel more comfortable to the patients as the advocacy group will be able to raise patient concerns with the management of the secure unit.

Staff
Twenty-six staff (all nurses) out of a possible forty-five responded to the survey. Only 31 per cent of respondents had received training on ethnic and cultural awareness. Eighty-eight per cent of respondents either did not know if information on personal care, e.g. hair, skin and beauty products suitable for those with particular cultural or spiritual needs, was available or stated that no information was available. Prior to the audit, the information available was limited. Seventy per cent of respondents either did not know if there was information available on the wards regarding different faiths or stated that no information was available. A list of multidenominational leaders is available on the wards but the majority of staff were not aware of this. Sixty-six per cent of respondents did not know if information was available on dietary needs or stated that no information was available. There is a chart in both ward-based kitchens which gives details of catering for multicultural groups.

Implementation of this has been agreed with the catering services. The staff results show an obvious discrepancy with the patient results. Those staff that had received training on cultural awareness prior to the audit had been very motivated by it and undertook to achieve appropriate actions – e.g. the provision of appropriate care items and ensuring access to appropriate religious facilities. This may have improved services for individual patients and therefore impacted positively on the patient results.

A number of recommendations were made following this audit:

1.   All nursing staff are to attend study days on the needs of patients from an ethnic minority, especially with regard to their specific dietary, religious and personal care needs. The training programme is continuing and has been perceived as very successful.

2.   The audit highlighted a lack of knowledge and/or a lack of information being available to nurses. This information is particularly important when the patient is being assessed. All staff should be aware

of how to obtain the relevant information regarding specific spiritual, religious, dietary and personal care needs. A new document has been designed for dissemination to the wards, taken from a Broadmoor Hospital document and a Berkshire Health Commission document *Handbook on Ethnic Minority Issues* (1995). This document looks at promoting a culture-sensitive service at the Unit and includes information about the dietary and personal care needs of many different religious and ethnic groups.

3. Standards were needed on the dietary needs and personal care of patients and on anti-discriminatory training. These have now been written. They ensure the provision of appropriate personal care which is sensitive to the specific requirements of all patients from ethnic and minority groups.

The standards mean that patients are provided with specific requirements appropriate to their personal care and hygiene and are meant to ensure that staff deliver culturally sensitive care within the Unit's policies.

It was noted in the audit that the restriction imposed by being a medium secure unit means that sometimes patients do not have the appropriate leave status in order to attend a specific place of worship. This is something that the multidisciplinary team has become more aware of recently. In these situations the appropriate religious leader is invited to the Unit to see the patient if that is what they wish. The Unit is too small to provide an area that can be used specifically for religious services. However, a quiet room can always be provided and all patients have their own rooms and this makes it easier for patients to observe any necessary religious practices.

CONCLUSION

The process described has not been easy. The Unit is still at the stage of developing services and in no way feels itself an expert in this area. The importance of the audit and the training package in developing services cannot be emphasised enough. Nor can the involvement of black advocacy and voluntary groups. Their input into the training programme has been of particular importance and their involvement continues to be encouraged. What is described in this chapter is a very practical and managerial approach to the development of services. It is not an easy area to develop.

The senior nurse has taken responsibility for ensuring the achievement of most of the above. She is from a white middle-class background and can feel uncomfortable teaching about racism and the development of services for black and other ethnic minority users. Addressing the beliefs and attitudes of others can also be very difficult, though very necessary.

FUTURE ACTION

Future action includes the continuation of the training programme and a further audit within six months, following another two series' of study days to ensure an improvement in staff knowledge. It is also necessary to audit the patients regularly to ensure that their needs are continuing to be met. It is possible that a black advocate group will be asked to undertake this audit to allow the patients to make as honest replies as possible.

It has been agreed that a small stock of appropriate personal care items for those from an ethnic minority – e.g. moisturiser and hair care products – are kept for admissions from prisons.

The high population of patients from ethnic minorities in medium security means there is a great necessity to develop services for these groups. The process described above is only the beginning of this development. It is recognised there is still a long way to go.

CHAPTER 17

Measuring Progress and Improving Quality

Jane Mackenzie and Carol Morgan-Clark

BACKGROUND

When the NHS was established in 1948, care and services were provided to meet the health needs of the indigenous population. Over the past 50 years, however, the composition and health needs of the indigenous population have changed significantly.

Previous health policies have done little to respond to the changing needs of ethnic minority patients and research has shown that this population has a worse health experience than the majority white population.

The increase in ethnic minority populations has put additional demands on the NHS to provide care which is culturally acceptable, is cost and clinically effective and which meets the high quality standards of holistic health care expected in the modern NHS.

In mental health services, there is clear and growing evidence of inappropriate admissions, poor pathways of care and service provision and treatment programmes that do not meet the cultural and racial needs of the ethnic minority population.

In addition, there is clear evidence that black people and members of ethnic minority groups experience institutional racism within public services, e.g. the police and the army, and, sadly, mental health services within the NHS are no exception.

The concept of measuring progress and improving quality in healthcare is not new but has been explicitly reinforced within *A First Class Service – Quality in the New NHS* (NHS Executive 1998). This document defines a framework for clinical governance that incorporates explicit, measurable standards of care and service, based on evidence that can be monitored regularly and improved where standards are not being met.

To measure the quality of healthcare provision within Broadmoor Health Authority, race and culture standards and audit programmes, standards for the provision of women's services, national and local patients' charters and a robust complaints management system all actively contribute to the measurement of achievement and progress. In all these areas there is a clear and specific focus on race and culture.

RACE AND CULTURE STANDARDS/AUDIT

A small, multidisciplinary race and culture working group developed a set of standards which were subsequently implemented in the hospital. An audit tool was also developed by the group and group members undertook training in the audit process prior to carrying out a hospital-wide audit. Standards monitored in the audit included:

- staff awareness of the Equal Opportunities policy
- staff awareness and level of implementation of the Race and Culture Standards
- level of race and culture training undertaken by staff
- information relevant to race and culture issues provided being available to patients and staff
- awareness of diet and cultural requirements when serving meals
- assessing staff awareness of the procedure for obtaining specific make-up and hygiene products for patients
- assessing staff awareness of the procedure for patients wishing to access religious facilities and spiritual advisers
- ensuring assessment of patients' cultural and racial needs and requirements has been carried out.

The first audit outcome identified significant deficits, but enabled us to focus on what and where the problem areas were. Action plans were then developed and demonstrable improvements have since been made. Further audits continue to monitor standards and focus on improvements in these and other areas.

PATIENTS' CHARTER

A local patients' Charter has been developed at Broadmoor Hospital, reflecting the national Charter (Department of Health 1996b) and the Mental Health Users Charter (Department of Health 1997a). Whilst not specifically developed to meet the needs of ethnic minority patients, the standards reflect some race and culture issues, but moreover focus on individual rights and expectations for all patients. In the monitoring process, specific racial and cultural issues are raised with individual patients.

The Broadmoor Hospital Authority Patients' Charter incorporates standards and explicit measurement criteria, some of which are listed below:

Courtesy, dignity and respect

- We will not discriminate against you on grounds of gender, colour, ethnic origin, nationality, disability, sexual preference or age.
- We will respect your cultural and religious beliefs.

Information and communication

- You will be provided with clear information that is easily understood.
- If English is not your first language, we will provide interpreter services for you.

Care and treatment

- You will receive a comprehensive multidisciplinary assessment of your needs and the most appropriate treatment to meet your needs, compatible with your cultural and spiritual beliefs.

The audit methodology for measuring progress in achieving these standards incorporates explicit criteria and comprises observation, checking records, looking at notice boards and availability of other information and, of course, asking patients and staff for their views.

Again, action plans are formulated as a result of the audit, and these continue to be monitored and improved where relevant.

STANDARDS FOR THE PROVISION OF WOMEN'S SERVICES

A set of standards specifically for women's services were developed by the Working Group for Women Service Users in Forensic Psychiatry, comprising community nurses and managers of women's services from Broadmoor Hospital, medium secure units and the private sector. In liaison with the Quality Improvement Service, the standards were formalised and an audit tool was outlined.

A process of implementation and an audit programme has been agreed, to measure and monitor progress of the standards within women's services.

Deficits identified will form the basis of action plans, which will provide the focus for improvement and perhaps further audit activity.

Standards include:

- the facility for women-only groups and activities to occur weekly as a minimum
- availability of a female GP on request, and a female nurse being available on each shift on women's wards
- women-only toilet and bathing facilities will be provided
- gender-sensitive training provided for all staff

- provision of a range of free female hygiene products for women service users.

COMPLAINTS AS PART OF THE QUALITY IMPROVEMENT PROCESS

Complaints are integral to the quality improvement process at Broadmoor Hospital Authority. This was further reinforced through the introduction of the *NHS Complaints Procedure* (Department of Health 1996a), combining the Quality and Complaints Departments and developing a comprehensive local policy for complaints. Complaints with a racial and cultural element, as all complaints, are taken very seriously and dealt with thoroughly and sensitively. Recommendations for change and improvement are again implemented and monitored. In addition, hospital-wide themes and trends of complaints identified are acted on and actions taken to change practice, deal with problems and prevent similar situations occurring.

Examples of complaints made and actions taken:

- Patient complains he was made to undertake a security search when he should have been attending the Mosque.

  Recommendation and improvements made: All wards have been formally required to prioritise search and other security requirements to occur at times that will enable patients to pursue their religious and cultural commitments.

- Patient complains of insensitive attitudes of staff and lack of cultural understanding.

  Recommendation and improvements made: Race and culture information packages have been revised and their importance and availability to staff reiterated. Cultural and racial sensitivity has been reinforced through the management process. Training programmes have been revised to incorporate real issues arising from the complaint and form part of individual staff training and development programmes. Where relevant, individual staff are identified to attend the 'Working With Difference' course as part of their personal and professional development programme.

- Patient complains of poor choice and variety of food relating to ethnic minority groups of patients.

  Recommendation and improvements made: The hospital catering manager regularly holds catering surgeries on each ward to deal with issues that arise. In addition, individual patients regularly meet with the catering manager and participate in devising specific diets and menus for vegans, vegetarians and ethnic minority groups. This has resulted in zero complaints about food consistently over a long period of time.

- Patients not able to access a variety of beauty and grooming products for ethnic groups.

Recommendation and improvements made: Standards relating specifically to this issue have been developed and are now monitored as part of a regular audit programme. Regular complaints reports and comparative data are provided, specifically identifying complaints from ethnic minority groups. This enables managers and clinicians to focus on and take further actions on issues of concern for these groups.

HOSPITAL QUALITY STANDARDS

Key areas are identified and prioritised for action each year. Information from these key areas is regularly collated and a formal reporting process is in place:

- *Seclusion and levels of observation* Monitoring of seclusion and levels of observation, using both qualitative and quantitative data, incorporates information reflecting gender and ethnicity.
- *Equal opportunities policy* Monitoring of the implementation of the Equal Opportunities policy is reported on regularly.

LISTENING AND ACTING ON USER VIEWS

- *Patients' Council* The hospital has an active Patients' Council, comprising representatives from a wide range of race and cultural backgrounds, and provides patients with the opportunity to raise areas of importance and concern. The Patients' Council meets regularly with key managers and clinicians within the organisation and are able to express their views. Their views ultimately contribute to and can influence the change and decision-making process within the hospital.
- *Women's Group* A women's group has been initiated to ensure women have the opportunity to raise issues of importance or concern to them in a safe and non-threatening environment.
- *Patients' Visitors/Relative Group* A visitors/relative group ensures relatives and visitors have the opportunity to meet regularly with managers and clinicians to voice their views and influence change, raise issues of importance and to access information about the hospital.

CLINICAL AUDIT

Clinical audit is a valuable tool for evaluating clinical practice. It interfaces with the broader quality monitoring process – which is very good at highlighting trends – by taking a more in-depth look at routine information. The methodology of clinical audit allows data to be analysed statistically, which suggests that the guesswork and poorly constructed opinions can be taken out of the interpretation of data, and also uncovers information which would otherwise not be available. One example within Broadmoor Hospital is the clinical audit work that has been undertaken around the topic of seclusion by ethnicity.

In 1995 a multidisciplinary group, known as SMARG (Seclusion Monitoring and Review Group), was set up to monitor seclusion. SMARG were concerned that there was a perception that ethnic minority patients were secluded more than white patients. Indeed, looking at the raw data it appeared that more black patients experienced seclusion, that their seclusion episodes were longer in duration and occurred more frequently than those of white patients. SMARG therefore decided to undertake a clinical audit project which would include a statistical analysis of the figures, to see if there was any significant difference in the way black and white patients were treated with regard to seclusion practices. The group initially wanted to look at seclusion rates for the different ethnic groups on one of the special care wards. However, it was difficult to draw any conclusions from the results as the number of patients in each ethnic group was so small. SMARG then decided to look at the seclusion rates for the different ethnic groups throughout the hospital.

Seclusion data were collected for the period 1 April to 30 June 1995. The raw data indicated that although 79 per cent of the patients in Broadmoor Hospital were white, they accounted for only 65 per cent of seclusions. The black patients (21% of the total) accounted for 35 per cent of seclusions. However, these overall figures do not take into consideration the numbers of patients who experience seclusion in each ethnic group. Further analysis was undertaken on the raw data in order to take this into account. Findings showed that only 13 per cent of white patients experienced a seclusion episode during this period compared with 20 per cent of black patients. On average a seclusion episode for a white patient lasted for 47 minutes compared with 71 minutes for a black patient. Of those patients who did experience seclusion, white patients had an average of two episodes each and black patients had an average of three episodes each.

In-depth statistical analysis was then carried out. This showed that there was no significant difference between seclusion rates for different ethnic groupings overall. However, as a subgroup, young (under 35 years) black males were over-represented in seclusion rates.

These findings were widely disseminated throughout the hospital in order to raise awareness of the issues at ward level. Clinical teams were requested to discuss these findings at their clinical team meetings. A summary of the project and findings was reported in the *Clinical Audit Newsletter*, which is widely distributed to all disciplines and levels of staff throughout the hospital. Various training events were held, both formal and informal, to raise awareness of the issues and to encourage actions for improvement.

A re-audit was conducted in 1997 in order to establish whether there had been any change in the situation from two years previously. Overall there was a drop in the proportion of patients secluded, from 14 per cent in 1995 to 11 per cent in 1997. In 1997, 72 per cent of patients secluded were white and 28 per cent were ethnic minority patients compared with 79 per cent and 21 per cent in 1995, respectively. Eighty-five per cent of seclusion hours were attributable to white patients and 15 per cent to ethnic minority patients in 1997, compared with 61 per cent for white patients and 39 per cent for ethnic minority patients in 1995 (Figure 18.1).

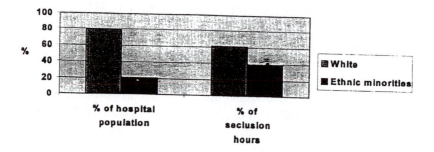

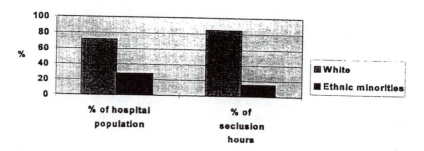

Figure 18.1

When patients were considered as a proportion of their ethnic group, 10 per cent of white patients and 14 per cent of ethnic minority patients experienced seclusion in 1997, a drop from previous levels of 13 per cent and 20 per cent respectively, in 1995 (Figure 18.2).

Secluded white patients had an average of 2 episodes in 1997, the same as in 1995. Secluded ethnic minority patients averaged 1.3 episodes in 1997 compared with an average of 3 episodes in 1995 (Figure 18.3).

Percentage of ethnic group experiencing seclusion

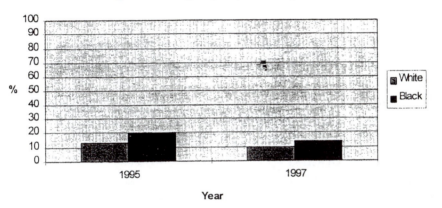

Figure 18.2

Overall there was no statistically significant difference in the pattern of seclusion for ethnic minority patients and white patients in 1997.

To summarise, this clinical audit project has shown that the overall rates of seclusion had decreased over the two-year period. Moreover, the rates decreased more for ethnic minority patients than for white patients. This had the effect of eliminating the statistically significant difference in seclusion rates for young black patients that had been present in 1995.

It would be impossible to attribute this improvement solely to the activities that resulted from the initial audit, as there may be other confounding factors

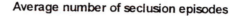

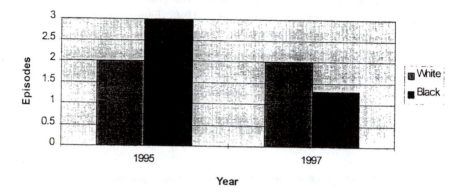

Figure 18.3

that have contributed. However, the situation undoubtedly improved over the two-year period, following a concerted effort throughout the hospital to raise awareness of the issues highlighted by the audit project.

MEASURING SUCCESS

Many problems and difficulties experienced within the hospital, on the whole, reflect the racial and cultural issues of those in society. At Broadmoor Hospital, being a comparatively small organisation, we are well placed to focus on identifying needs for change and improvement, and to ultimately raise standards.

To make it happen and to demonstrate success, firm commitment and support from the Hospital Board and senior managers needs to be visible. In addition, clear and explicit standards and robust monitoring and audit systems are essential. An open and honest culture is paramount, where people are treated with respect and equity and where easily accessible and fair complaints systems are welcomed, as a way of positively improving the service. It is important that patients are listened to, their voices heard and concerns and issues of importance are acted on.

Dynamic training and development programmes for individual staff should be ongoing, where continuous learning is implicit and research and evidence-based practice is not just something the library sends around on their monthly update list. At Broadmoor Hospital, we believe we have come a long way in achieving many of these success criteria. We cannot, however, rest on our laurels and it is only through continuous and ongoing measurement of progress that we will ensure that an implicit culture exists reflecting high quality, secure forensic psychiatric services which really do 'provide equity and non-discrimination to all our patients, regardless of race, culture, gender, age, sexual preference or disability' (Broadmoor Hospital 1998b).

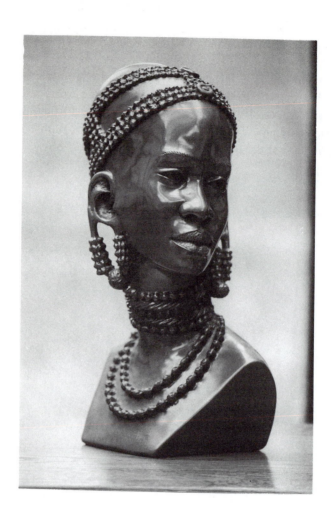

Head of Zulu woman

CHAPTER 18

Translating a Vision into Reality
Broadmoor's Partnership with ACMHA
Elaine Elvey

INTRODUCTION

The Mental Health Act Commission (1995) reported its concern in its 1993–95 report about the long delays in transferring patients identified by clinical teams as suitable for discharge into less secure conditions or community facilities. The report cited difficulties as being 'patchy provision at local level' and 'very little preparation' to enable the client group to achieve successful 're-habilitation' into 'society, community' and home.

'Patchy provision' (the Commission's words) and lack of preparation forms part of the overall problem of inconsistency of care. In addition, the ongoing poor communication within and across the various sectors continue to exacerbate this problem. Patchy provision and abysmal communication across the various statutory sectors is certainly part and parcel of our experience at local level, particularly in trying to co-ordinate services around individuals who were discharged back into the community to live in semi-independent or independent living conditions.

It is with this mirrored concept in mind that the preparation (through befriending), rehabilitation and reintegration (through socialisation, education and re-skilling) scheme was born. This concept also keenly matched the philosophy of ACMHA which shaped the holistic services with which the organisation already worked.

It might be useful at this juncture to provide the reader with an overview of ACMHA's philosophy and approach to its work with people of African and Caribbean descent. The organisation's approach is based on a philosophy which is underpinned by the fundamental concept of black psychology, which relates to the inter-relationship between mind, body and spirit. This approach facilitates the exercising of personal choices through a process which affirms the client's ability, while simultaneously facilitating the development of the client's potential.

In effect, it recognises that some understanding of the whole person is critical to the type of service and the form delivery of that service takes. This is particularly true within the arena of mental health.

Holism is therefore a symbol of ACMHA's approach to working with our communities, be they within or outside the mental health sphere. 'Holism' at its simplest, means treating the patient's symptom not in isolation but as part of a total health profile. This is applicable whether the service in question is therapy, advocacy or that of co-ordinating a range of services around the individual from which one intends the client to benefit. In so doing, a wide range of information about the client, his or her circumstances, preferences and state of mind contributes ultimately to the final result. It is also the recognition that the client or patient is an individual and has a traditionally holistic attitude to treatments.

The system in its existing form and orientation still does not acknowledge that a great many of its charges are people who are intelligent and articulate. The aim of the existing treatment regime should be to return such individuals to a state of wellness, responsibility, self-esteem and independence. We derive our independence from having identifiable markers in our daily lives: study, work, employment, family and friends. For the detained of African and Caribbean origin, the opportunity to experience and benefit from most of the above was never provided.

It is therefore from this abiding philosophy that the programme of befriending, rehabilitation and reintegration was conceived. The programme, which first commenced with befriending, began in 1996 as a pilot scheme at Broadmoor Hospital.

We were keenly aware of a number of cases where families automatically distanced themselves from these clients. Culturally there was a great deal of stigma attached to having a relative in a psychiatric institution. The stigma felt by African and Caribbean families was directly related to the way in which the mentally ill were seen and treated in Europe – in particular the black mentally ill, who are nearly always represented as axe-wielding murderers or rapists. The stigma and social embarrassment for such families far outweighed any level of commitment they may have had to maintaining links with the individuals concerned.

Distancing themselves was also made a great deal easier by the ludicrous practice which is part and parcel of a system which continues to send people to medium and high security facilities hundreds of miles away from their communities.

It was this complete removal from the reality of everyday life, removal from everyday contact and social activities and removal from social functioning which so decreased the social skills of such individuals, thus posing the most serious problems on discharge.

We were soon to learn, once the programme had begun, the extent to which even the most articulate of our clients had lost any real understanding of the dynamics of friendship and social relationships. Providing links, therefore, with individuals from the same culture, and developing those links along the lines of friendship, seemed and was indeed the first step.

This chapter will show why such a scheme came about, the design of the scheme, who the key players are and what the programme intends to achieve. It is also part of the overall plan that the programme will be evaluated once the first group of clients have moved through all three parts of the programme.

THE CONCEPT OF 'PREPARATION (BEFRIENDING), REHABILITATION AND REINTEGRATION'

It is generally agreed that at least 35–50 per cent of those detained in high security hospitals would be better served in facilities of lower security. However, it cannot be denied that high security settings and, latterly, private secure units boast the kind of educational facilities which allow those detained to gain skills which settings of lesser security only dream of. Educational programmes are usually in abundance – art and craft facilities, gymnasium, the opportunity to learn skills in carpentry, catering and light engineering. Whether such facilities are being used to significantly contribute to rehabilitating the more receptive detainees is questionable.

The preparation (through befriending), reintegration and rehabilitation project is designed to provide practical, psychological and social skills, as well as support to those who are due to be discharged from any of the three high security hospitals, first to a medium secure unit and eventually back out into society. The main aim of the project is to set up the mechanisms required to co-ordinate and make the best use of the various individuals and agencies who are involved in the existing care, development and treatment of this client group.

The primary aim is to provide clients with the necessary skills – educational, employment and social – *before* they are returned to society.

Naturally it is recognised that this will not happen in its entirety before a number of individuals have been discharged. The emphasis, however, is placed on the fact that there should be some understanding that this work needs to commence some considerable time prior to discharge. The expectation therefore is that clients prepared in this way will, in the long term, actually feel they have a stake in the society to which they are being returned. They will not feel automatically inclined to behave like long-term dependents, but as contributors and participants.

The concept of working to prepare clients who are likely to be discharged sooner rather than later, whilst also providing a *befriending* service, was discussed with the DOH in 1997. Discussions and proposal for the befriending service commenced with John King of the Social Work department and Chandra Ghosh in 1995.

All concepts are influenced by present and historical factors. The concept for this programme is deeply influenced by the recurring themes of:

- the revolving door syndrome which is usually precipitated by the reality of
- loneliness and isolation for those returned to a community into which they no longer fit, as well as being totally
- ill-prepared to manage some of the most basic aspects of everyday life, together with
- no personal links and very tenuous agency links in the community to which they have been returned.

ACMHA was keen to ensure, therefore, that these themes remained central to the design and development of the programme.

THE PROJECT

The project in its simplest form would act as a bridge linking the special hospital, medium secure unit, locality practitioners, employers and education institutions as the client moved from one setting to the next. This was designed with the aim of providing a service that would ultimately rehabilitate and reintegrate those individuals of African and Caribbean origin, currently detained at Broadmoor, who chose to join the programme – the emphasis being on choice.

The service would involve the key practitioners at Broadmoor at the stage of plan development and implementation. Practitioners from the other sectors would be involved at different stages of implementation at the earliest. This was to be carried out through a process of ongoing communication, update and monitoring.

All participants in the programme would be involved in the construction of their own 'development plan'. Unlike the care plan, the development plan would contain practical and achievable objectives which would have some real impact on how they reconstructed their lives back in society.

The plan aimed to take on board re-skilling of those clients who possibly had a trade or career before entering the system, with a view to developing employable skills. Or alternatively, the plan aimed to incorporate the client's educational interest, with a strong emphasis on this leading to qualifications either at college or university. From our experience, we knew that some clients had an interest in pursuing a particular course of study, which on completion could lead to gainful employment. In a number of cases, unfortunately, this interest was neither being used as an aid to the overall treatment process nor as a goal-orientated objective.

A great deal of the programme would involve pinpointing these interests and ambitions from the outset, ensuring that all the practitioners involved had access to the development plan, and providing the necessary support which would allow the client to work towards achievable goals. Each client's development plan would therefore form the basis of their programme.

Before the operation could commence, however, the groundwork of selling the idea to purchasers and practitioners alike needed to be done. It is important to note that from the outset a partnership and commitment to the project was forged between ACMHA and Broadmoor Social Work department, led by John King. There were numerous telephone calls and meetings, which is an inevitable part of establishing any project.

As far as we were aware this was going to be the first project of its kind. Here was a project that would not only seek to befriend individuals whilst detained in high security hospitals, but provide them with a service that would gear them up towards identifying future goals for themselves whilst their befriender moved through the system with them. This would perhaps be their first opportunity at committing themselves to working towards this, as part of an entire developmental process.

Those individuals who made the commitment and signed up to the programme would need to understand that they had a stake in their future, and would be taking on part of the responsibility of contributing towards their own development.

From the outset the befriending relationship was key to the rest of the programme. The befriending contact would serve to engage the client in a trusting working relationship. It would also serve as a channel through which the ingredients needed for the rehabilitation and reintegration package would be collected. It was also going to serve as the springboard from which one would construct the other stages of the programme on a client-by-client basis. Most important of all, it was agreed that possibly for the first time the lead for constructing what went into the client's development plan would come from the individual client concerned.

Securing genuine commitment from all those involved was paramount, as this was destined to have a great impact on the functioning and viability of the programme.

As far as ACMHA was concerned, this was pioneering a new way of working with clients from the African and Caribbean communities.

PROJECT DESIGN AND PLAN

Purchasers, practitioners and stakeholders needed to be informed about the whole project. This entailed presentation of the proposed project to a number of different individuals and groups.

The project design as presented to the various individuals and groups consisted of three phases:

Phase 1 Befriending and preparation

- Assessment, matching, befriending/mentoring and familiarisation
- Cultural contact
- Identifying and building relationships with key practitioners within the hospital
- Identifying and building relationships with key practitioners and purchasers at medium secure unit and local level.

Phase 2 Rehabilitation and reintegration

- Identifying skills, educational interests and level of support needed
- Training
- Identifying appropriate therapeutic support
- Identifying key practitioners
- Identifying possible employment opportunities
- Monitoring progress.

Phase 3 Reintegration and resocialisation

- Identifying and interacting with social activities
- Training
- Recognising and understanding acceptable social practices and behaviour
- Branching out
- Monitoring progress.

Phase 1 of the project was established through the befriending service, which has the advantage of being able to operate as an independent project but can also work equally well as part of the rehabilitation and reintegration programme.

As stated earlier, befrienders would establish the cultural link whilst providing low-key social preparation and interaction. This we felt would be as valuable for those individuals for whom discharge was not part of the immediate plan (1–2 years), as well as for those who were likely to be discharged within the next couple of years.

Whilst assessing those clients who signed up to the programme, it became clear that a number of potential clients were so institutionalised that only the befriending part of the service would be of long-term benefit to them. Nevertheless, it was agreed that the option would be made available to them to join the remainder of the programme, should their level of social functioning and interaction improve. We felt it would be possible to pick up changes, positive or negative, through supervision of the matched befriender and periodic case review and assessment.

Our presentation of the programme consisted of a project plan which outlined the various steps:

Step 1 — Present the project to key purchasers, practitioners and other identified stakeholders.

Step 2 — Identify and assess clients who wish to join the programme.

— Create client's development plan. Identify relevant practitioners who will be involved with clients who are closest to being moved on.

Step 3 — Identify and meet with medium secure unit practitioners to discuss move-on facilities.

Step 4 — Identify and meet with employers re: employment and work placements.

— Identify and meet with colleges re: course requirements where clients indicate the need to continue studies.

Step 5 — Identify and liaise with community social worker and community team.

— Identify and liaise with GP.

— Identify and assist in re-establishing other social links at local level.

THE TEAM

The staff team to support the project was set at seven people: a team of social workers, the co-ordinator for volunteers, the education and employment officer and an administrator. We also envisaged working with a member of the probation service, possibly by phase 2 of the project.

In an ideal situation where funds were not an issue we at ACMHA would have wished the project to be led jointly by a senior social worker and probation officer. It soon became clear that this would not be possible. We were therefore happy to proceed with the senior social worker as lead practitioner at ACMHA, as this was felt to be the most appropriate person. We also felt that at Broadmoor, and indeed at medium secure facilities, the social work practitioner should be the lead person with whom we would liaise and develop further plans.

In a number of cases it was our experience that the more informed social worker often knew how to access key information about subsidiary services, both within their own locality and in other boroughs and in some cases other parts of the country. But at least they knew the mechanisms to operate in order to gain the required information.

The knowledge base of the social workers on the team, would need to include not only key information about the workings of the psychiatric system but also the workings of the wider mental health system nationally.

At this point attention needs to be drawn to the geographical spread of the project we set out to tackle. Current practice for placing clients in medium secure and high security institutions is 'bed-led'. Individuals are placed in facilities based more on availability, and far less on whether the facility is appropriate for their treatment and rehabilitation. As a result of this, our existing client list consists of individuals who are from the north, the southeast and the west of England. There was a much greater concentration from the south of England, but the main point is that this project was going to operate on a national scale.

NATIONAL AND GEOGRAPHICAL OPERATION

By the second year of the project, work of a national nature had commenced in southern England, in London. Two clients who had spent just under one year on the befriending scheme had already moved on. Not as we would have liked, with a full development plan in place, but given that we are London-based, and had already presented the programme and made some of the necessary links with at least one of the medium secure units, it was encouraging.

A presentation to not only key members of staff but all staff on the unit in question followed fairly soon after. The social worker on the unit was identified as the link person and lead person for the programme on the medium secure unit. This was a positive sign. Phase 2 had finally begun in the south of England. The response from the staff on the unit was positive and there was a very good spirit and atmosphere in which to work.

Managing the programme nationally involved dividing the team into geographical areas, where each social worker would have responsibility for a particular area. Two of our three remaining social workers were due to join the team in 1999, which would give us five of our seven personnel. Our move-on list currently shows a further four clients. This we anticipate would happen towards the end of 1999.

All social workers involved knew initially that their job would involve a significant amount of travelling to units and locality services within their allocated geographical area. But they also knew that, possibly for the first time, they were being asked to draw on all their experience, communication skills and negotiating skills to make such a project work.

CONCLUSION

I hope this chapter has given the reader a picture of the project and how it has unfolded thus far. What I hope this pioneering idea conveys is the need to be open and receptive to new ways of working with those individuals who occupy the forensic area of the psychiatric system.

A number of clients who have signed up to the programme began their journey through the criminal justice system at an early age. In some cases some are still struggling with the stark reality of how an index offence, which would have given them four years in prison, turned into 12 years or more.

In trying to construct this programme we examined the social climate which existed at the time, and how this contributed to not all, but some of the more bizarre and unjust cases which found their way to Broadmoor. In our opinion, fortunately, depending on one's perspective, a number of these cases are predominantly men in their early thirties and mid-forties. There are also a handful of women, some with young children, which the programme recognises it must address in a somewhat different way. These are still largely young people.

This programme will require significant funding over the next 2–3 years, but if commitment as shown in phase 1 is sustained throughout, then society and the public purse will ultimately have made an enormous saving.

As explained earlier, the project is based on linking and co-ordinating the various practitioners who at differing levels will have some involvement in providing services to those clients who have elected to enter the programme. A key contact person was identified on both sides. At Broadmoor we were very fortunate to have as our link person John King whose commitment and enthusiasm matched our own. The chief co-ordinator long-term from ACMHA was earmarked as either the social worker or probation officer, but in the interim the role was being facilitated by the co-ordinator for volunteers. This fitted into the scheme of things rather well, given that the first stage involved a great deal of communication, training and organising those volunteers who would be on the programme. The contact person at ACMHA for stage one and the first steps was the main co-ordinator for volunteers. The chief co-ordinator for the programme as a whole would be ACMHA's chief social worker.

This was the first programme of its kind and it was wonderful to experience this level of commitment on both sides. Charting development and progress at every stage was also possible as both ACMHA and Broadmoor shared a belief in the programme and a willingness to see it succeed.

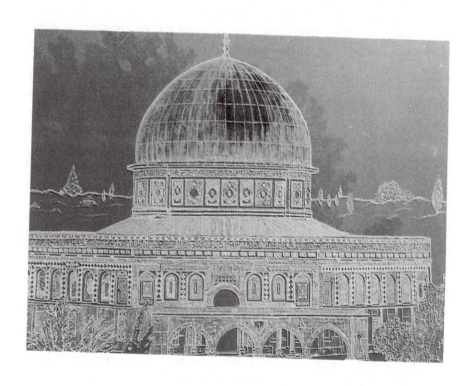

Dome of the Rock, Jerusalem glass engraving – Nizar Boga

CHAPTER 19

Meeting the Spiritual Needs of Muslim Patients

Nizar Boga

THE RELIGION OF ISLAM

Adhered to and practised by over one billion Muslims in the world, the religion of Islam today forms the second largest faith in Great Britain after Christianity. The population of Muslims in Britain at close to two million comprises almost all nationalities of the world. It is also the fastest growing religion not only by natural birth but also through a sustained programme of conversion. It is inevitable that the public institutions generally would correspondingly have growing numbers of Muslims whose needs and requirements have to be addressed in the climate of equal opportunity and fair treatment.

It is a well-known concept in Islam that the health of the body and mind is a necessity for physical existence as well as a prerequisite to the spiritual well-being of the soul. A troubled mind in particular becomes a factor which impacts on the individual's ability to comprehend one's actions and this leads to the person not being able to pursue his religious beliefs. In Islam, although such persons are not held responsible for their actions nor open to criticism for neglecting their religious duties, the society is duty bound to provide relevant welfare service to meet their specific needs. Indeed, such persons ought to be helped in any form or manner as part of a community care service for the fulfilment of a religious requirement.

It is for this reason that Prophet Muhammad taught that a Muslim in his/her prayer should include a request for good health emphasising that no other supplication is more pleasing to God (TIRMIDHI). He is reputed to have said that to possess a healthy body and sound self and an assured provision is like owning the whole world (TIRMIDHI). Such is the emphasis laid on good health in the Islamic faith. Correspondingly, therefore, anything that mars the achievement of good health is discouraged and indeed forbidden, e.g. eating of unwholesome food, smoking, partaking of intoxicants, taking illicit drugs and even over-eating itself (NISAI and TIRMIDHI). Equally true is the fact that when the body or mind is affected by factors outside one's control, the community would offer help, particularly in matters of faith and beliefs.

Generally speaking, the main issues involved in fulfilling the needs of Muslim patients are as follows.

Identity and recognition

Muslims will readily declare their faith even if they are lapsed or non-practising. It is therefore important to recognise and then address their special and sometimes sensitive needs, particularly in secured settings where the trappings of the institution may not be particularly friendly or obliging.

Prayers

Prayer five times a day is compulsory for every Muslim person. The prayer is preceded by an ablution or bath. On Fridays the midday communal prayer is perhaps the weekly landmark for most Muslims. Friday does not become a Sabbath but a time to meet and reflect in the mosques. It is essential, therefore, that not only the facility is provided, but in special hospitals and other places of secure settings regular arrangements are made for patients to be brought to the place of worship at the time appointed. The sermons and prayers are led by the Imam whose duty is to encourage and persuade as many patients as possible to attend. The Imam also takes the opportunity after the prayers to advise the attendants on various aspects of the religion. While in the mosque, patients may wish to consult the Imam on personal matters. This is often facilitated by the Imam being able to visit the wards to see the patients who were not able to attend the prayers, guiding and helping them overcome some of their worries and anxieties. Where the Imam feels that the hospital authority could make more effort to improve the facilities and/or arrangements there should be an access route, perhaps initially through the chaplaincy. The Imam can also assist with the provision of funds from outside sources to meet specific needs of the patients, e.g. study fees. Indeed, this has happened twice in Broadmoor Hospital. It is therefore important to have a specifically provided prayer house or mosque where patients can feel more relaxed and cared for. The prayer house or the mosque should be of adequate size with fitted carpet and have a provision for toilet and making of the ablution. Again Broadmoor Hospital has taken the lead recently by refurbishing a detached building in a central location and allocating it for Muslim patients.

While the mosque is normally open for Friday prayers, one ought not to forget that it is also a place for the five daily prayers. Although on these occasions the Imam would not be present, there is no reason why the prayers cannot be led by one of the Muslim patients. The visiting Imam will ensure that adequate training is given to those who wish to volunteer. However, the difficulty in providing an escort facility should not be minimised. Muslim patients are, in the circumstances, advised and encouraged to perform their prayers individually in their rooms.

Friday Prayer is a compulsory act of worship requiring devotees to leave their trade and business in order to attend the mosque. The prayer is held at mosques at midday. It is preceded by a sermon that is partly on religious observances and partly on current affairs affecting the lives of the Muslims. In special hospital it is proper that the sermons reflect the patients' predicament and how they can derive personal comfort and spiritual assurances.

In this respect, areas such as health, anger, forgiveness, communal harmony, patience, good manners, life Here and Hereafter, religious injunctions, prayers, etc. are covered and would be considered as beneficial. Along with this, the reading of the Holy Quran and other Islamic books are highly encouraged.

Muslims are also required to celebrate their two annual festivals of Eid with special prayers. The Hospital Authority should make arrangements for patients to participate in the prayers followed by a feast that the Imam could undertake to be brought for the special occasion. It is also necessary that patients are not forced to carry out normal work on these days.

The mosque in Broadmoor Hospital already has the facility to stock necessary books and copies of the Quran which are also distributed to the patients.

Fasting

Fasting during the month of Ramadan is compulsory for all Muslims who are adult and not otherwise constrained because of illness or health condition requiring medication during the day. The fast is between dawn and sunset. It requires complete abstention from any food, drink or smoking. Prior to the commencement of the fast, a light meal is taken. The hospital authority therefore needs to make facilities available for this as well as for the main meal to be taken after sunset. The Imam can demonstrate his willingness to spend longer hours with the patients and share meals with them at the break of fast once or twice during the month. Taking of the meals by the Muslim patients outside the normal meals time is a critical issue that needs to be addressed seriously.

Food/drink

Lawful or Halal food is a must for Muslim patients. This can either be cooked in the hospital or brought from outside. It is also important to ensure that a variety of food is purchased in order for the patients not to feel isolated or in any way marginalised. It is true that a vegetarian diet is a substitute for Halal food but this must remain a choice rather than a replacement. Of course, pork and pork products are strictly forbidden. Where, therefore, food is cooked inside the hospital, staff need to be trained to ensure there is no cross-contact with pork or other unlawful food. The Imam can assist in the training as well as in giving general advice to staff and patients. Muslim patients should ensure that they have registered their request for Halal food.

Similarly, alcohol is forbidden and again caution is necessary where food is prepared. It is also important that the staff are sympathetic to the food being brought from outside by the relatives or the Imam. Indeed, the staff must provide facilities for it to be received, stored and served at the appropriate time.

Registration

Muslim patients must be asked to register with the hospital Chaplain so that in the event of death or other incidents, their wishes can be complied with or respected – funeral rites, special prayers in case of grave illness, communication with relatives, etc. It is also important to ensure that the patient's family is kept informed in order to avoid any misunderstanding in the future.

About three years ago, Broadmoor Hospital was faced with an incident where a premature death of a converted Muslim patient required a very sensitive negotiation with the deceased family. On the one hand there were the expressed wishes of the deceased and on the other the hospital had to deal with the demands of his relatives. The Chaplain played a major part and with the help from the Imam he managed to contain the problem. The Imam eventually arranged the funeral through a mosque.

RELIGIOUS DISCRIMINATION

Special hospitals and places of secure setting need to have far more serious consideration in dealing with the spiritual needs of the minority religions. The rules of the establishment ought to safeguard sensitivity, and a mechanism should be in place to deal with friction among patients and between patients and staff. Although racial equality is provided for in the Race Relations Act, religious discrimination is not, even though it can impact much more on the minds and hearts of the victims. Bullying and victimisation can be tempting for all concerned. In the setting in which the patients find themselves, unpleasant incidents and perhaps misunderstood statements can leave a long-lasting sour feeling between individuals.

Although the climate of Islamaphobia, which the Runnymede Trust has recently highlighted in its report, applies to all aspects of life in Britain, its impact in special hospitals can lead to explosive situations with perhaps incalculable consequences.

Needless to say, staff training ought to incorporate not only traditional areas of equality and equal treatment but also a religious dimension so that Islam is understood better and in a positive light. Here again the Imam can assist with staff training and participate in patient counselling. The benefit can be mutual between the patients, staff and the hospital authority in general.

SECURITY CHECKS

It is understandable that hospitals may have to carry out some checks including physical checks on the patients, for security and other reasons. What needs to be borne in mind is that a Muslim woman has to wear, at all times, a full dress from the neck to the ankle and also completely cover her hair unless she is in the company of her husband or other close male relatives or other females. She has also to be seen by a female doctor. For the same reason when a search is made of her person, although it is considered unpleasant and reprehensible, she would be advised to co-operate providing the persons carrying out the exercise are female and provided there is minimum exposure of her body.

For male patients, the minimum body coverage required is from navel to below the knees. Exposure and inspection of the private parts, unless done for medical reasons, is considered objectionable. However, compliance with the law and rules of the establishment needs to be considered and the patient would be advised to co-operate providing the search is made by male staff, is not unduly prolonged and there is no other acceptable alternative to the method employed.

The Imam has had to give similar advice to a patient recently in Broadmoor. In case of doubt or misunderstanding by the staff or the patients, the Imam should be available to give advice and help.

PATIENTS' NEEDS

It is one of the Islamic principles enshrined in the saying of Prophet Muhammad that Muslims should relieve a person's anxiety and meet his or her needs wherever possible.

Patients in special hospitals will often talk about their worries, their confinement, family matters, health problems and even about their relations with other patients. They are also often dependent upon the staff for their immediate concerns. For their spiritual needs, they would usually wait until they see the Imam, who would perhaps visit on Fridays.

The Imam, however, should be available for contact at home at any time when an urgent need arises. This is done through the staff making the initial telephone call and the patient then being allowed to speak with him either in the presence of the staff or privately if necessary. Broadmoor Hospital already facilitates this arrangement.

A joint approach between the Imam and the Chaplain to explain certain aspects of religious requirements is sometimes necessary and can be beneficial. Broadmoor Hospital has had one such case that was dealt with expeditiously to the benefit of all concerned.

With the consent of the Imam, patients can be given his address to write to. The Imam in Broadmoor Hospital has also in the past arranged for a patient subsequently transferred to a less secure setting to visit a local mosque for a Friday communal prayer. An example such as this makes the existing patients feel confident about the establishment in which they live and also assured of the community support when needed.

CONTACT WITH PATIENT'S FAMILY

In Islam family plays a pivotal role in the conduct of life. In some cultures, extended family structure also ensures that more than just parents are available to seek help from. When it comes to fulfilling the spiritual needs of the patient, often the patient's family will seek help and guidance from an Imam. It is not unknown for the family to contact the Imam who is known to the patient. This would work to the advantage of the whole family as there would be continuity of service and would help build more confidence in the system established in special hospitals. The help in this case can also include relieving financial difficulties, family differences and disputes, etc. The hospital authority, therefore, needs to assist patients in this respect and recognise the Imam's role.

CONCLUDING OBSERVATIONS

Much of what has been said is against the background that, compared with Christians, Muslims have a much stronger bond with their religion and family. This is evidenced in the proliferation of mosques and community centres, both purpose built and adapted buildings, throughout the United Kingdom. The religious practices are not reserved for weekly attendance at the mosques. Prayers five times a day, a whole month of fasting in a year and eagerness to study the Holy Quran both inside the mosques and at home are perhaps examples of the spiritual needs of a Muslim. The non-separation between religion and state makes it compelling upon Muslims to consider religious practices as fulfilling a whole way of life. However, like most religions the detailed knowledge of Islam would appear to be beyond the reach of many. As religious practices depend on knowledge, classes, lectures and conferences are usually held to assist those who wish to pursue their faith in earnest. In special hospitals, such opportunity perhaps may not exist. However, the hospital authority may wish to consider this as an extension to the existing facilities.

It is often seen in institutions of this kind that there is domination of one particular religious denomination. This is becoming more and more unacceptable. In multi-ethnic Britain with varied religions and faiths, Muslims as well as others should have a voice at the centre. There must be awareness programmes and training for staff and patients. The hospital authorities should arrange occasional meetings of the Chaplains, Imams and ministers of other faiths in order to discuss common patterns of service provision and its responsiveness, and share knowledge and experiences. They should then work towards producing a more informed and equal service to the patients, particularly in a secured environment where confinement is for long periods and where patients would find more time to reflect upon their beliefs, their religious requirements, their place in society and their future. Given this facility, and nurtured possibly by the presence of their religious advisors – in Islam the Imam – there is a possibility that it might have a therapeutic effect on their lives sufficient to rehabilitate or change their personality to the benefit of the community at large.

A Trader

A trader of African Arts and Crafts
At 3rd world currency the whole world laughs
But carry on and sell your wares
Of masks and Abyssinian jewellery
Economical gifts we all should share
Not just political skulduggery.

This was me and I was this
A trader's life is full of bliss
The pound, the yuan and the mark
Selling and Selling I made my mark
Not foreseeing the evil waiting in the dark
Calculated, premeditated the seal of the devil
Jaws of the shark.

They pounced when I was in my prime
Not guilty...still made to do my time
When in the belly of the beast
The voices 'oh Lord' they did not cease.

The madness and uncertainty
The medicine brutality
But then he came to set me free
The power of the Trinity

The Holy Ghost, the lion also the lamb
The evil could not understand
The light had conquered the dark for now
And let me trade my wares somehow.

Anthony Roach

CHAPTER 20

The Experience of Being a Black Patient

My first encounter with the psychiatric system was after being arrested for a series of serious offences. I was 20 years old, bewildered, confused and disturbed. My father had died some months prior to the beginning of my series of offences. At the time of my father's death I had sought help from the authorities to come to terms with my grief and cope with the responsibility of bringing up my younger siblings. Although I did meet with the social services, they said they were unable to offer us any assistance other than inadequate benefits. The year was 1981 and I opted for a life on the crime-ridden streets of London in order to ensure that my responsibilities vis-à-vis my younger siblings was discharged. This lifestyle eventually led to my capture two years later, for a string of armed robberies.

Angry, bewildered, confused and disturbed, still suffering from what I now know was a grief reaction to my father's death two years previously, I was now facing the might of the British judicial system. I was sitting in front of a man who tells me he is a psychiatrist sent by the authorities to determine whether I am mentally fit to stand trial. I can't be mad – I'm not prepared to entertain the notion that I might just have mental health problems, so I tell the psychiatrist, in as forceful a way as possible, to get lost. Even if the psychiatrist had told me more about mental illness I would never have accepted that I could possibly be mentally ill. I just saw myself as an angry young man who had to do something about helping to bring up his younger siblings.

However, I was sent for trial despite displaying classic symptoms of a paranoid illness. 'After all, all black men are criminals aren't they?' 'Lock them up and throw away the key,' as a newspaper headline at the time proclaimed. 'One nig nog less on the streets the better,' said the judge at an after-dinner speech, again reported in the *Sun* newspaper. From then on it was not difficult for me to realise where I was in the racial divide.

Consequently, instead of receiving treatment for a severe paranoid schizo-affective illness I found myself languishing in a category 'A' prison cell serving multiple life sentences. For three months I was in solitary confinement on 'good order and discipline' (GOAD) where I could not contact any other inmates and only had hostile conversations with the prison warders who constantly hurled racial abuse. They even engaged in physically pushing and shoving me whenever they wished. On two occasions I fought back and was placed in the 'strong box', which is a specially designed cell within a cell. These strong boxes are designed to bring down the body temperature rapidly, thus incapacitating you by bringing on a hypothermic-like state, which is made all the more disconcerting by the total deprivation of natural light.

Although I was 5ft 8 inches tall, I only weighed about eight-and-a-half stones at the time. I believe my food was regularly tampered with and I was being given sedating substances. The prison warders always ensured that they had enough of them to overpower me whenever I gave any indication that I was going to resist. On reflection, this to me was another example of the notion that a black man is strong and always needs more warders to be restrained.

One day, after a particularly eventful week of many hostile verbal exchanges between myself and the prison warders, I returned to my cell after taking my allotted hour's exercise to find the outline of a body drawn on my mattress with red ink marks simulating blood and boot marks, all around the head area. The message was clear – they wanted me to believe they intended to harm me. On noticing this I immediately started banging frantically on the door and screaming abuse at the prison warders. The governor of the prison happened to be visiting the segregation unit at that moment and asked for me to be brought before him so he could ascertain why I was making such a manic racket. I was brought before him in his office, which was around the corner from the segregation unit, and proceeded to tell him about the body drawn on my mattress and the clear threat it implied. At that point the governor said he did not think his warders would be capable of doing such a thing but he offered to come and have a look with me at the offending mattress.

When we reached the cell I pushed open the door gesticulating animatedly but I was amazed to find that my original mattress with the outline of the body on it and the red ink representing blood had gone and in its place was an untampered clean mattress. I could not think straight. I knew that obviously the prison warders had done something to replace my original mattress, which only made me even angrier and more animated. It took me many years to work out that the cells either side of my cell were empty and the prison warders must have swapped one of those mattresses for the tampered one. All this made me seem mad. I started wondering whether I was losing my mind, until one night in the depths of darkest despair overwhelmed with suicidal thoughts I eventually tried to take my own life. Fortunately my bid failed. Unbeknown to me I was on a list of vulnerable prisoners and I was on a 15-minute watch.

I was forcibly medicated and transferred from one prison to the hospital wing of another prison. Months later the Medical Officer decided that I needed to be in a psychiatric hospital and not in prison so I was duly transferred to Broadmoor in an extremely paranoid and disturbed state.

Within my first hour of being in Broadmoor Hospital any illusions I had of making a fresh start and of not being racially abused, bullied or intimidated by those entrusted with caring for me were shattered as I was put through the well-rehearsed admission process. This admission process was intended to dispossess me of any last vestige of hope or dignity that remained and involved being stripped naked in front of six burly nurses and placed in a bath containing roughly four inches of yellowy orange water. Two of the nurses crowded in close and put their feet on the rim of the bath, leaning menacingly over me. They told me that they could deal with any 'hard nuts' that come from the prison system and if I stepped out of line I'd be dealt with. I was later to find out to my cost that this was no idle boast or threat. I was also later to find out from other patients that I had had a relatively easy admission process because the charge nurse in charge on the day of my admission was considered a liberal minded fair man who frowned upon the excesses of some of his staff, so they had been somewhat constrained. This was borne out by the fact that although I only had four inches of bath water, it was lukewarm and not freezing cold, as was regularly inflicted on new admissions by one particular acting charge nurse when he was on duty and in charge. I quickly realised that there was little if any consistency between the different nursing shifts. What was permissible under one charge nurse might lead to being secluded (being stripped and placed in a room with no access to windows or fresh air) or, even worse, being placed on large doses of Largactil under another charge nurse on a different shift. Largactil was the much feared and infamous 'liquid cosh'. It was often used in a punitive way with varying doses depending on your misdemeanour. I was placed on 200 milligrams of Largactil (forte suspension) four times a day for telling one member of staff to treat me with respect, after he had spoken to me in a manner which I found offensive.

I quickly gained a reputation for being 'a black smart-arse', to quote one member of staff's description of me, and a management problem despite never resorting to any form of violence. For a number of years I was placed on a high dependency ward, medicated and given no access to therapeutic interventions such as psychology. I was 'stitched up' (had evidence fabricated against me) and sent to the intensive care wards as a warning to others in case they dared to challenge the racist regime that was operating openly. During this period my attitude towards the staff hardened because of the liberties that were being taken with me. At this time I was also unable to work on the initial mental health problems that had led to me being in hospital because I was unable to trust the staff who were supposed to be caring for me and facilitating my treatment.

During this time I regularly took cannabis to relieve the stress and tensions which I felt. Since I could not trust the staff to treat my illness or treat me fairly I had to look within myself to find the resilience to regain my sanity and maintain my integrity and dignity as a black man.

How can we as vulnerable mentally disordered offenders learn to tackle and change our unacceptable behaviour when those that are entrusted with our welfare do not discharge their responsibilities professionally and allow their own prejudices to influence their attitudes and behaviour?

Around the end of the 1980s a new management structure was introduced to Broadmoor with the remit of changing the antiquated, draconian, inherently racist culture that had been allowed to grow and fester virtually unchecked, resulting in the deaths of a number of young black men within the institution.

The new management gradually started having some success in combating the excesses of the most unprofessional staff by a combination of disciplinary measures and education. Those staff who still insisted on behaving unprofessionally were politely asked to find alternative employment elsewhere. During this time many of the 'dinosaurs' left the hospital. However, many remained but with their power to behave in discriminatory ways much diminished. It took a few years for this enlightened approach to filter down to ward level but eventually we (the patients) started reaping the benefits of anti-discriminatory policies and an enlightened approach.

I was placed on a progressive ward where I was given access to therapy. Although the therapy was not culture-sensitive, it did however give me the opportunity to explore all aspects of myself, my attitudes towards life and in particular my attitudes towards my offending behaviour. Through a mixture of individual one-to-one therapy with extremely enlightened psychologists, which proved very challenging, and group therapy work I was able to come to terms with many aspects of my personality which I had previously avoided. Through this therapeutic work I was also able to establish contact with my principal victim.

Broadmoor is no longer an insular environment. Today many groups and bodies have been given access to us and cater for the many diverse needs of the black population in Broadmoor. The influx of a new breed of highly motivated, totally dedicated enlightened professionals has done much to rid the institution of its worst elements. However, the remnants of this particular group have become insidiously cunning, camouflaging and disguising themselves amongst the new breed of dedicated professionals by keeping their unacceptable attitudes covert amongst their ever-decreasing circle.

As we approach the millennium I suppose the challenge is, how to prevent any black patient now and in the future from having to endure the indignity of racial discrimination in whatever form. Whilst it has been possible to curb the excesses of certain racist staff through the introduction of policies and the threat of disciplinary action, it has not been possible to curb the behaviour of those racist patients who use racist abuse safe in the knowledge that they face no censure. After all, how do you legislate against attitude?

The battle is far from over. There is still much work that needs to be done to improve the quality of life for black and ethnic minority patients in Broadmoor. But with new initiatives such as culture-sensitive psychology with black psychologists and groups run specifically for black patients for us to explore ourselves without the Eurocentric slant we are gradually gaining ground.

By recognising our cultural and religious needs the authorities have gone a long way towards equalising service provision. However, I believe that there is still a long way to go and perhaps it is necessary to listen to the individual no matter how angry he or she may become. The fact is that many black patients have a lot to offer in terms of their experiences but I feel they don't get heard or adequately understood because they express themselves angrily or find it difficult to articulate their frustrations at the racism they encounter.

Broadmoor Hospital has embarked on a challenging journey and there will be occasions when initiatives to promote a sensitive service will be thwarted and sabotaged, but I am optimistic that with an ever-increasing contemporary workforce this journey will prove to be positive for all future service users.

CHAPTER 21

Awareness and Change

A Training Initiative at Broadmoor Hospital

Charles Kaye

PRACTICAL STEPS

As each individual's views are shaped by the cultural context, it is necessary for students to explore their own beliefs and values. This requires the use of experiential teaching and learning methods, enabling the exploration of feelings and clarification of partly formed concepts, the challenging of established notions and the exploration of ethics and morals in relation to culture and ethnicity. Le Var (1998).

In recognising the existence of cultural dissonance between many ethnic minority patients and their mainly white carers, Broadmoor Hospital has started a programme of education, awareness and understanding entitled 'Working with Difference'. Its key aims are:

- To equip staff with a repertoire of skills and appropriate knowledge for effective mental health patient care.
- To enable professionals to reflect on their practice and to facilitate new ways of working with differences and diversity.

The programme takes the form of ten days' learning, a day a week spread over ten weeks. The modules include lectures on all aspects of race and culture, practical exercises, short placements with other organisations, projects rooted in the work situation and discussions centring around patients and their experiences.

The first course was held in the autumn of 1997 and the second, six months later. Those attending were as shown in Table 2.1.

Table 2.1 Attendees at Broadmoor Hospital's 'Working With Difference' courses

Role	First course		Second course	
	Broadmoor Hospital	Other employers*	Broadmoor Hospital	Other employers+
Nurses	15	4	10	4
Rehabilitation staff	2		1	
Social work		1		
Advocacy				1
Complaints			1	
Security			1	
Total	22		18	
From ethnic minority background	5		6	
	* local authority (1) other special hospital (1) medium secure unit (2) mental health trust (1)		+ prison service (1) other special hospital (1) medium secure unit (1) mental health trust (2)	

All sessions were held at Broadmoor Hospital. Three months after the end of the course, a follow-up day was held to review progress.

With regard to staff it has to be noted, with regret, that no doctors or psychologists and only one senior manager attended a course. Seniority and status does not confer omniscience, nor does it absolve those individuals from learning. The latent nature of what we sought to explore makes it likely that it will rest unperceived at all levels of institutions and agencies.

OBJECTIVES AND GAINS

In other words, how well do we truly understand Aboriginal peoples: their behaviour, their culture, their spirituality, their values? I grew up in Manitoba and my views were influenced by what I saw – severe alcohol dependence, poverty, low levels of education, stories of violence. My impressions of Indian people were clearly prejudiced by the negatives – I can't really recall the positives.

Gerry Cowie, Canadian Correctional Service (1992)

Why did people come on the course? The participants in the second course put forward their individual initial objectives:

- to evaluate advances in practice
- to understand the 'totality' of needs
- to heighten awareness ('open mind')
- to influence strategy in terms of operational issues
- to develop a platform for race and culture
- to promote service equity
- to improve knowledge and practice
- to improve service for Muslim patients
- to gain an educational experience
- to maximise staff expertise and effectiveness
- to share knowledge.

Some individuals had very specific objectives in mind: producing policies, influencing their organisations. Others had been dragooned into the course, 'chosen' by their manager in an arbitrary fashion. As with any course, enthusiasm and 'stickability' varied; some individuals missed sessions and some had to respond to emergencies at their workplace to the detriment of their attendance. Overall, commitment and willingness to learn were impressive; and the work on practical projects in their work areas echoes this.

Learning was very visible. There was an initial exercise which reviewed, in a very practical sense, the use of language: acceptable and unacceptable terms. This in itself revealed unwitting insults, ignorance and real disagreement. A group session with a black psychotherapist began to explore self, the awareness of difference and the existence of prejudice. A range of formal lectures included epidemiology, historical development, legal framework, religions, anthropological and cultural studies, institutional racism, and the everyday practice of psychiatrists. The personal experience of patients was also shared.

The mixture of ethnic backgrounds among the students (and the lecturers and course directors) added considerable savour to the proceedings, sharpening many of the challenges in discussion.

What did students gain? Here are some of their own comments:

Made me think about what I say and how I talk.

Made me think about language.

I question things I see on the ward.

I'm learning from the group itself: views and feelings. I'm still working with that.

It's a disparate group: it challenges attitudes I had (particularly re: poverty and class).

It's changed my attitude; given me insight into the Black African Caribbean patients on my ward.

The make-up of the group is a good balance. I discuss with an open mind.

I now stop and realise the groups I used to place people in.

I've learnt about the historical development of forensic psychiatry.

It troubles me that I might say things, through ignorance, that are wrong!

What did students agree to pursue? Here are some of the projects they chose to take on:

- Translating/interpreting – a directory.
- Identifying 'black' organisations in the local community. Establishing links, facilities, services into the Unit; and for patients going out.
- 'Language' – increase staff awareness: nurses and what they say.
- Support network for black women patients (related to abuse histories)
- Create links with local community organisations. Befriending scheme.
- Use of language.
- Support group for black staff in hospital.
- Activities for black patients.
- Patients attending the mosque: influence on their behaviour, making other staff aware of this.
- Training in awareness of ethnicity; audit.
- Analysis of needs of patients from North African background ('others'): examination of services/support available.

Particularly noteworthy was one medium secure unit which had a senior nurse on one course and a deputy on the next as part of the unit's determination to improve its services relating to ethnic minority patients.

For Broadmoor Hospital in particular there is now a small cohort of staff who can begin to influence their colleagues and actively help to change views and attitudes in the hospital.

CONCLUSIONS

Cultural barriers have been cited rather too glibly to explain the serious difficulties which exist in providing acceptable services for ethnic minority populations. A much more important factor is, to put it bluntly, racism. Though sometimes overt, racism is usually covert, but it is deeply ingrained in professional and institutional practices. Most often it is totally unconscious and goes unrecognised by staff and service users (Murphy 1991)

It is clear from the briefest survey of contemporary life in the agencies and institutions of this country that racism and prejudice, overt or covert, exists towards ethnic minorities. What is open and above ground in its expression can be challenged by law: across the nation, and by policy within each institution. What is covert, subterranean, or even internalised to the degree that it is not even recognised as prejudice, is much more difficult to combat. Fiat will not work in that context; where the majority have institutional power, the unseen bias will continue to operate against disadvantaged minorities, helping in the process to ensure they remain disadvantaged, below.

There must be policies and guidelines; the flags must be seen to wave publicly. But that is a mere beginning. In order to change behaviour and create insight and understanding, there is an urgent need for education and encouragement. This has to take place in a safe environment where staff can explore the emotional, intellectual and social aspects of difference outside the pressure of the work and beyond the scepticism of their colleagues.

As with most real learning, the discovery of self will precede the acknowledgement of others' needs and demands. It may seem strange to have to state this in the world of psychiatry where such essential observations should be commonplace, but we have to be aware that, carers or not, professionals or not, we remain part of that society where the fleck of prejudice runs consistently and dramatically through out basic fabric. The difference is that our responsibility is greater given the task we undertake.

Two courses will not change a national service, or even a single institution. A determination to recognise the need to *change practice* to alter the way in which individuals relate, has to be the starting point. These two courses described, and other related initiatives, represent the concerted effort of one institution to begin the process of change. The biggest challenge is to maintain the impetus so that staff and patients feel that they can challenge prejudice, explore difference and develop a better understanding. That is the start of the journey.

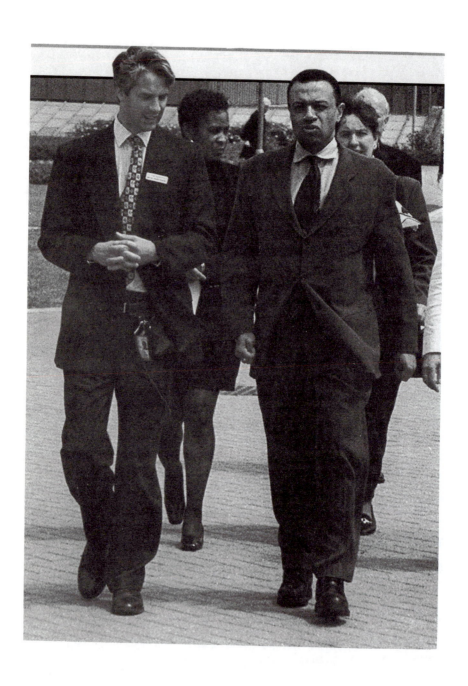

Paul Boateng visits Broadmoor Hospital

CHAPTER 22

Progress in Broadmoor Hospital

Tony Lingiah

There is extensive evidence of the negative effects of individual and institutional racism experienced by members of minority ethnic groups and yet it is a fundamental value of the National Health Service that it should meet the needs of all sections of the community equally. Providing the same service in the face of differing need does not give an equitable service.

The high security hospitals – Ashworth, Rampton and Broadmoor – have for several years now made attempts to address the needs of ethnic minority patients and have frequently engaged in discussions about the need to provide services in a culturally sensitive manner. Several policy documents have been written, but it seems that the impact on service delivery has changed little and both patients and relatives from ethnic minority groups perceive the services on offer as anything but culturally sensitive.

The late 1990s witnessed a surge of interest in minority issues and under the NHS Executive's equal opportunities unit the health issues and service provision for black and other ethnic minority patients acquired a sharper focus on the agenda. The implementation of mandatory ethnic monitoring for all in-patients in England from 1995 created a meaningful framework for health authorities to demonstrate service planning which reflects the population being served.

This chapter will explore practical approaches in the delivery of an equitable service to patients from black and ethnic minority groups at Broadmoor Hospital in a forensic setting.

WHO ARE WE TALKING ABOUT?

It should be emphasised that terms such as 'black', 'race' and 'ethnicity' have all been favoured or rejected at different times and in different contexts and that there is no universally accepted phraseology. The term 'black and ethnic minority' is used for preference throughout this chapter to underline the common experience of patients from these groups and in no way minimises the diversity of language, culture and religion which exists within the minority groups themselves and which can be significant in influencing health and access to health services. The term 'African-Caribbean' is used to refer to people of Caribbean origin.

BROADMOOR HOSPITAL

Broadmoor Hospital, one of three high security facilities in England, provides specialist healthcare and treatment for men and women with a mental illness or personality disorder, who require the services of skilled professional staff in a safe and secure environment. The hospital provides a full range of treatment for its patients including assessment, speciality care and rehabilitation. The service revolves around its 22 wards (16 male and 6 female) which have all been refurbished and now provide a comfortable environment for patients.

As a provider of high security services, Broadmoor Hospital has a contract with a single purchaser, the High Security Psychiatric Services Commissioning Board (HSPSCB). Under the contract with the HSPSCB the hospital provides 443 occupied beds – 88 for women and 335 for men. Patients from ethnic minorities make up approximately 25 per cent of whom 15 per cent come from an African-Caribbean background. Broadmoor Hospital serves a wide catchment area including counties and localities as diverse as Devon, Lewisham and Oxfordshire. With a staff complement in excess of 1250, of whom 8.4 per cent are from black and ethnic minority background, the hospital's total income for 1997/98 was in the region of £42 million.

Race and culture issues were brought into sharp focus by the publication of an enquiry report entitled *Big, Black and Dangerous* – looking into the circumstances surrounding the death of Orville Blackwood, a young African-Caribbean patient at the hospital in 1991 – which concluded that: 'Management and staff alike need to recognise that there are differences and these differences need to be catered for' (Prins *et al.* 1993, p.55)

Race and culture issues have now become very prominent in the planning and delivering of psychiatric services and Broadmoor Hospital sought to engage in a range of initiatives to ensure that the services offered reflected and respected cultural sensitivity and was delivered with a high degree of professionalism.

The High Security Psychiatric Services Commissioning Board, as the purchaser of services, were under no illusion that a clearer focus about service equity issues needed to be achieved and a robust framework was established in their 1996/97 contract which to a large extent was prescriptive. This probably reflected the need to engage, as a matter of priority, in outcome-related initiatives on issues of service provision for patients from ethnic minorities at the hospital.

Broadmoor Hospital Authority acknowledged that there were gaps in the services and used the HSPSCB standards to launch a fresh start to service equity issues. The appointment of a professional development and equal opportunities adviser (himself from an ethnic minority background) with responsibility for service equity issues became a component of the equal opportunities strategy.

To enable the hospital to deliver on the contract, a comprehensive framework was established which would translate strategic objectives into operational service delivery. The following formed part of the framework.

Equal Opportunities group

This group was set up to lead on the key initiatives of the Equal Opportunities Strategy. It consisted of both clinicians and managers and is chaired by the Director of Human Resources. An incremental approach was adopted in relation to implementations of initiatives and a realistic timetable, prioritising key initiatives, was endorsed by the group. Close monitoring of progress in relation to implementation was undertaken by members with an annual report of the Executive Board.

Training

Staff training on issues of race, culture and psychiatric management became central to the development of the equal opportunities framework. Three levels of training have been implemented at Broadmoor Hospital, namely:

1. *Promoting a culture-sensitive service* (induction course) All new entrants to Broadmoor Hospital receive, as part of the three-week induction course, a presentation on issues relating to service delivery to patients from ethnic minorities, professional responsibilities and attitudes and the hospital's expectations of a quality service. Inductees are encouraged to explore key concepts relating to stereotyping, institutional racism and anti-racist behaviour.

2. *Working with Difference. The practitioner, the patient and the service* This is an innovative 10-day course, available annually, which focuses on key themes of race, culture, ethnicity and the psychiatric service.

    Formal presentations included in the training relate to historical developments, epidemiological trends, legislative framework, religious, anthropological and cultural issues, use of language, institutional racism and concepts of a culture-competent psychiatric service.

    The conscious process of acknowledging difference (occasionally a painful process) is a fundamental theme throughout the course. Once participants have gained confidence and are comfortable with the material, the focus changes to practical projects to enable learning that takes place to be translated into actual initiatives which will impact on the quality of life of patients.

Examples of projects initiated by course participants include:
* developing core service standards
* setting up a befriending scheme for African-Caribbean patients
* links with local black community organisations
* a support group for black staff in hospital
* a support network for black women patients.

One key lesson learned by the course organisers was the need for closer involvement of the relevant manager or sponsor. The work-based projects were designed to encourage participants to apply what they were learning to their clinical practice, but success was mixed; some projects thrived, while others experienced organisational blockage.

(c)   *One-day mandatory training on cultural awareness* Broadmoor Hospital Executive Board have now made a commitment to a full-day workshop for all staff on issues of race and culture. This rolling programme planned for delivery over the next 18 months will capture the essential elements of what is needed to promote a culture-sensitive and a culture-competent service. Central to the training materials will be the analysis of scenarios of real events and the exploration of personal values and beliefs which shape our attitudes to ethnic minority groups. The workshop aims to create greater awareness of cultural differences and essential skills needed to deliver on the needs of ethnic minority groups.

The three levels of training currently available create the capacity to promote greater awareness of race and culture issues and the potential for staff to maximise their contributions and support to contemporary practice in the area of equal opportunities.

Core service standards

As part of its commitment to promote the development of services which are more culturally sensitive for black and minority patients, Broadmoor Hospital Authority established a framework for the implementation of a set of formal race and culture standards across the hospital. A small working group was set up comprising of doctors, nurses and managers to develop core service standards on:

- Equity in service delivery   Appendix 1
- Anti-discriminatory training   Appendix 2
- Diet   Appendix 3
- Personal care   Appendix 4
- Religious and spiritual needs   Appendix 5

All the standards have now been implemented throughout the hospital. A rigorous audit tool has been developed to monitor implementation.

Appointment of a black psychotherapist

For some time, the hospital authorities had been concerned about the inequity which existed in relation to the lack of opportunities for black patients to engage in psychotherapeutic interventions. The reasons for this are multifaceted and undeniably complex, but as a hospital we were determined to have in place a more satisfactory arrangement which would demonstrate our commitment to a more equitable service in this area. The Authority contracted the services of a well established black psychotherapist/counsellor to provide a bespoke service for black patients. The initiative, on its first year review, has been successful on two levels:

- The black psychotherapist was perceived to be a positive role model for black patients.
- The cultural background of the black therapist enabled dynamics relating the culture, race and ethnicity to be explored in a more focused manner which facilitated the establishment of a clearer cultural identity for patients. Some patients who have in the past been perceived as 'difficult to manage' responded positively to psychotherapy in that they felt that they were better understood and began to engage with issues which had not been previously discussed.

The initiative is to be further developed to enable other black service users to benefit from this service. In addition, a co-therapist, from the black community, has now been appointed to further enhance the service. Our long-term aim is to have an integrated service which is needs-led and is culture-sensitive and it is felt that the current initiative will minimise the damage done by the lack of early interventions for black patients.

Living with Diversity group

Community living can be stressful and impersonal. This could be further compounded in a high security environment which imposes a high degree of control on movements. To add to this, the psychopathology of mental illness can turn a simple interaction into a complex relational conflict. Several of the wards at Broadmoor Hospital have a patient population with diverse ethnicity and diagnosis, and attitudes and language from some patients leave a lot to be desired. The 'Living with Diversity' group was set up to promote greater cultural awareness. Its aims and intended outcomes are:

- *Aims*

– To establish a forum for patients to explore issues of race and diversity in the context of communal living.

– To further enhance awareness of cultural differences.

- *Intended outcomes*

– To promote greater awareness about cultural differences.

– To enable group members to develop an empathic approach to cultural diversity.

– To promote greater understanding of the experiences of being 'different'.

The group is made up of approximately ten patients from both the majority white and ethnic minority population and has fortnightly meetings lasting for an hour. The general principles of group work are adhered to and it is facilitated by two nurses. The subject themes relate to race, culture and ethnicity and issues surrounding attitudes, behaviour and the use of language. The material discussed can trigger off arguments which need to be sensitively managed, but group members are encouraged to confront anti-social language and behaviour. The impact of this initiative needs to be evaluated, but generally there is support for such a group from both patients and staff. We believe that ultimately the 'Living with Diversity' initiative will contribute to combating prejudice, stereotyping, harassment and undignified behaviour in the clinical environment.

Resource pack on Cultural Diversity

Staff in direct patient care have a need for information which is easily accessible and is user-friendly. A resource pack has now been developed which contains useful information on issues of culture and race which enables staff to understand the needs of patients from ethnic minority backgrounds in their care. The hospital is committed to, and has responsibility for, ensuring that all care is delivered in a non-discriminatory way with a high degree of professionalism and it is hoped that the information presented in the resource pack will serve to enhance knowledge in this challenging area of work.

In brief, the resource pack contains information on the following key themes:

- Historical background to immigration
- Migration from the Indian subcontinent
- African-Caribbeans and migration patterns
- Promoting anti-racism and anti-racist healthcare

- Culture and customs
- Cross-cultural communication
- Communicating across a language barrier
- Different minority groups and specific issues relating to language, religion, food, practical care, blood transfusions, death and death rituals.

Staff comments about the resource pack have been positive and it is hoped that staff will refer to the material when caring for patients from ethnic minority groups to enable them to deliver a culture-sensitive service.

Setting up a spiritual service for Muslim patients

As a hospital, Broadmoor is committed to ensuring that patients of minority religious groups have the same right to practise their faith as those of the majority faith. The success of establishing a 'multifaith' platform at Broadmoor Hospital is attributed to the passionate quest for equity in spiritual care by our chaplain, who has tirelessly worked for this aim over the last fifteen years. There is a growing number of patients both from minority groups and the white population who follow the Muslim faith. The hospital recognised this need and has now provided a dedicated prayer area with supporting resources to enable regular observance of the Muslim faith. The hospital employs a part time Imam who co-ordinates spiritual support for Muslim patients with the help of two Muslim staff members. An inauguration ceremony took place in late 1998 for the 'da-ood Reedman's Mosque', named after the first patient who converted to Islam at Broadmoor Hospital. A successful framework has now been established for 'Friday prayers' conducted by the Imam, who also provides a service on the intensive care wards for patients too ill or disturbed to attend the mosque. There is now a population of approximately twenty patients of Muslim faith at the hospital and the service being offered has proved to be both spiritually enriching and 'therapeutically positive' for our Muslim patients. We have collaborated with external Muslim organisations who have donated prayer mats, copies of the Koran and other religious material. The IQRA Trust has been most supportive in our endeavour, and our wish for the future is to have more collaboration with Muslim communities for the benefit of our patients.

Patients' Equal Opportunities group

This group was set up to support the various initiatives introduced at the hospital and also to provide a platform for patients to discuss issues of equity in service delivery.

The aim of the group is:

To provide a forum for patients to raise issues relating to equal opportunities within the hospital. To further provide a means of solving the problems where possible or referring them to the most appropriate person within the hospital for resolution.

The group consists of a mixture of patients and staff representing views on ethnicity, race, gender and disability. The themes developed at the bi-monthly meetings range from issues of service delivery to staff attitudes, harassment, recruitment and training. Senior members of the hospital's executive board are invited to attend to discuss strategic issues and to provide progress reports on initiatives implemented.

The benefits of having such a group can be summed up on two levels:

- *Developmental* The patients attending have to conform to the protocol and criteria of a business meeting and the group provides a 'growth and development' opportunity. Additionally, they develop confidence in presenting their views and interfacing with senior members of staff in the organisation.

- *Operational* The patients feel that they have an opportunity to influence decision making on issues which impact on their life. The platform provides an 'undiluted' focus on live, real issues impacting on patients' quality of life for managers to engage with. In addition, the key themes discussed are fed back to the main equal opportunities group, which influences the planning and development of future equal opportunities at the hospital.

Cultural awareness theme days

Over the past few years, the hospital has been very keen to graduate cultural awareness through 'theme-days' activities, thus enabling both patients and staff to enhance their knowledge about different cultures. The most recent 'cultural theme' focused on Africa and a week-long calendar of activities was organised to reflect African art, music, history and food culminating in an 'African evening' when patients and staff attended an African musical programme followed by an authentic African meal. External voluntary organisations attended some of the activities and the feedback from patients has been very positive, which has encouraged the hospital to integrate 'cultural awareness' theme days in service planning and provision. Already plans are under way for a 'multicultural' theme week!

In addition to the initiatives described, there has been progress in some other areas, namely:

- A *cultural support group* has been set up for staff to explore issues of discrimination, harassment and prejudice. This group provides a platform for staff to discuss their experiences and to receive support and understanding in the validation of their feelings – regardless of whether the encounter was with staff or patients.

- A *complaints mediation service* has been set up for black patients, an initiative promoted by one of our team leaders to enable patients who are reluctant to lodge a formal complaint to have an opportunity to engage in informal discussions about the issue.
- *Skin, hair and beauty products* are now available in the hospital patients' shop, which enables black patients to purchase from a range of products specifically designed for them. In addition the hospital shop now stocks greeting cards with 'ethnic' motifs. Furthermore, the shop will honour any requisitions for products not available on the shelves by buying direct through their suppliers of ethnic products.
- A *befriending service* from the African-Caribbean Mental Health Association has been established for patients who do not receive any visitors. The hospital has contracted for a monthly service and currently fourteen patients benefit from this initiative. ACMHA has also organised summer activities and a yearly Christmas party for African-Caribbean patients. This has proved to be a very successful initiative for our patients and we are presently exploring the feasibility of extending the service to other black patients at the hospital.

One could argue that these initiatives should, in any case, be available in an integrated service, but in an ever-increasingly competitive NHS some priorities have better appeal than others, and service provision for ethnic minorities has not been on top of the agenda. With the best will in the world, unless Chief Executives have a passion for equal opportunities, service inequities will always be a reality.

Broadmoor Hospital has risen to the challenge it faces in the arena of equal opportunities and service equity and it would be apt to quote from the recent award Broadmoor Hospital won for its innovative focus on equal opportunities:

> Though changing attitudes in an institution such as Broadmoor – among patients as well as staff – is a colossal challenge, its ethnic minority patients have noted some remarkable changes thanks to this programme. It is valiantly ambitious, and though it has a long way still to go, the very active interest in it, from the top of the organisation augurs well.

As a hospital, Broadmoor is passionate in its pursuit for clinical excellence, and the evidence to date has been encouraging for what promises to be an exciting and rewarding journey.

APPENDIX 1
Service equity policy

1. *Statement*

    Broadmoor Hospital Authority is committed to providing services which are delivered sensitively and in a professional manner to all patients regardless of ethnic background, gender, disability, age, sexual orientation and respecting their religious and cultural beliefs.

2. *Purpose*

    The purpose of this Policy is to make explicit the Authority's approach and to identify ways in which the Hospital should take action to monitor inequalities in service provision and take the necessary action to reduce them.

3. *References*

    The Policy satisfies the requirements set out in the Patients' Charter, the Department of Health guidance on ethnic monitoring and the Race Relations Act 1976.

4. *Procedure*

    The Authority will foster a culture in which equity in service provision, quality and patient satisfaction is valued.

4.1. The Authority will provide clear information about services provided and develop core service standards in relation to ethnic minority issues.

4.2. The Authority will develop a framework to provide a translation service for patients who have specific language and cultural needs as far as resources allow.

4.3. The Authority will encourage patients to use the complaints procedure if they are not satisfied with the services provided.

4.4. The Authority will consult with users of services through 'focus' group and satisfaction surveys and establish links with voluntary groups representing ethnic views.

4.5. The Authority will provide focus training in regard to gender issues, cultural sensitivity, anti-discriminatory practice and transcultural communication.

4.6. The Authority will act swiftly in proven cases of discrimination and unprofessional behaviour in regard to patient care.

APPENDIX 2
Anti-discriminatory training

Standard Reference No: RCAR1

Hospital Reference No: 1

Topic: Race & Culture

Sub Topic: Anti-discriminatory Training

Care Group: All staff employed by Broadmoor Hospital Authority

Hospital Service Standard

Implement Standard by: 1998/99

Audit Standard by: 1998/99

Signature of Chief Executive:

Initiated by: The Race & Culture Group

Standard Statement

Broadmoor Hospital Authority is able to demonstrate that steps are in place to equip all staff to respond appropriately to the differing individual, social, cultural, religious and other needs of black and minority ethnic patients who we care for. This ongoing initiative will be implemented on the basis of a medium to long term objective.

Structure	Process	Outcome
1. An action plan is in place identifying training needs for all disciplines, which includes: – timetable of training – staff groups – training resources required. 2. A resource pack on 'cultural diversity' is available on all wards for reference. 3. All disciplines are aware of the Equal Opportunities Policy, Disciplinary Procedure and Codes of Conduct. 4. All disciplines are aware of the hospital's Philosophy and Purpose statement.	1. All new staff to the Hospital have access to training on 'Promoting a culture-sensitive service' during induction. 2. Key ward staff to attend 'Working With Difference' course and take a lead on ward training and service delivery issues re: ethnic minorities. 3. All staff adhere to 'service equity' policy and foster a culture-sensitive approach in the care of patients from minority groups. 4. As part of the hospital's Complaints Procedure a trends analysis is maintained on discriminatory practice.	1. All staff can demonstrate skills in caring for patients with social, cultural, religious and other ethnic minority needs. 2. Broadmoor Hospital Authority enforces the disciplinary procedure in proven cases of discrimination and acts swiftly and vigorously in any case of discrimination to patients.

AUDIT PROTOCOL

Audit Reference No: RCAR1   **Hospital Service Standard**

Hospital Reference No: 1

Audit objective: That processes are in place to equip all staff to respond appropriately to the differing individual, social, cultural, religious and other needs of black and minority ethnic patients.

Time frame: Initial audit to be completed within six months, thereafter on an annual basis.

Sample: All wards which are identified by the resident population of ethnic minority patients.

Auditors: Members of the Race & Culture Group   **Date:** 1998/99

[Target group]	Method	[Code]	Audit criteria
Ward noticeboards/ information folders	Observe	S2	Is information provided on all wards about cultural diversity?
Staff	Ask	S3	Are all disciplines aware of the Equal Opportunities Policy, Disciplinary Procedure and Codes of Conduct?
Ward noticeboards/ information folders	Observe	S4	Is there evidence of the hospital's Philosophy and Purpose statement?
Nursing process/ treatment plans	Chart audit	P3	Do staff maintain high professional standards when caring for patients with differing ethnic needs?
Staff	Ask		
Training records	Chart audit	P1 O2	Have all staff received anti-discriminatory training as part of their induction programme?
Staff	Ask		
Training records	Chart audit	P2 O1	Have key ward staff attended the 'Working With Difference' course?
Staff	Ask		
Training Records	Chart audit	P2 O1	Are training sessions facilitated on all wards to raise awareness?
Staff			
Complaint report	Chart audit	P4	Is an analysis of trends available on discriminatory practice?
Quality Improvement Service			

APPENDIX 3

Diet

Standard Reference No: RCAR2

Hospital Reference No: 2

Topic: Race & Culture

Sub Topic: Diet

Care Group: All patients being cared for by Broadmoor Hospital Authority

Hospital Service Standard

Implement Standard by: 1998/99

Audit Standard by: 1998/99

Signature of Chief Executive:

Initiated by: The Race & Culture Group

Standard Statement		
Broadmoor Hospital Authority is committed to providing all patients with a choice of menu that reflects religious, cultural and ethnic needs.		
Structure	Process	Outcome
1. Information is provided on the availability and provision of appropriate diets in the patients' admission information pack. 2. A master chart of religious/cultural and food 'Do's and Don'ts' is available on all wards and in the catering department. 3. Training is provided for all key staff groups who prepare and serve food, thereby raising awareness of religious and cultural significance. 4. A menu that provides genuine choice is provided. 5. Colour-coded serving utensils are provided. 6. A dietitian is available for consultation via referral.	1. On the patients' admission a thorough nursing assessment of cultural/religious dietary requirements is completed and documented and referred to the dietitian if needs are identified. 2. The Primary Nurse liaises with the patient and the catering department to ensure that choice is available appropriate to need. 3. At meal times staff are sensitive and adhere to religious, cultural and ethnic needs of patients, e.g. fasting, prayers, personal hygiene. 4. All precautions should be taken during the serving of meals to ensure there is no cross-mixing of food by using colour-coded serving utensils in the preparing and serving of food.	1. The meals provided meet the cultural/religious requirements of our service users. 2. Information is provided to patients and staff about diets appropriate to those patients having cultural/religious and ethnic needs. 3. All staff adhere to protocols in relation to respecting cultural and religious diversity.

AUDIT PROTOCOL

Audit Reference No: RCAR2   **Hospital Service Standard**

Hospital Reference No: 2

Audit objective: That all patients are provided with a choice of menu that reflects religious, cultural and ethnic needs.

Time frame: Initial audit to be completed within six months, thereafter on an annual basis.

Sample: All wards which are identified by the resident population of ethnic minority patients.

Auditors: Members of the Race & Culture Group   **Date:** 1998/99

Target group	Method	Code	Audit criteria
Patients	Ask	S1 P2	Are patients provided with information on the availability and provision of diets in the admission information pack?
Staff	Ask		
Information available	Observe		
Nursing process	Chart audit	P1	Is a thorough nursing assessment of cultural/religious dietary needs completed?
Noticeboards/ information folders	Observe	S2 O2	Is information available about diets appropriate to those patients having cultural/religious and ethnic needs?
Menus	Observe	S4	Does the menu provide genuine choice?
Staff	Observe serving of meals	P3 O3	Do staff adhere to religious/cultural and ethnic needs of patients at meal times?
Staff	Observe serving of meals	S5 P4 O3	Are precautions taken during the serving of meals to ensure there is no cross-mixing of food, e.g. use of colour-coded serving utensils?
Nursing process/ dietitian referral forms	Chart audit	S6 P1 O1	Are referrals to the dietitian documented if identified?

Catering for multi-cultural groups

This wall chart aims to provide information about differing religions and cultures. It offers practical suggestions to facilitate the serving of correct food to clients belonging to minority groups. It should be noted that individual variations may exist, therefore it is essential that an in-depth eating and drinking assessment is undertaken for each individual client prior to the planning of individual menus. All minority meals will be made available.

	UNITS	HINDUS	MUSLIMS	SIKHS
Specific cultural and religious requirements to be considered in the process of menu planning	EGGS	Possibly	Allowed	Probably
	MILK	Allowed	Allowed	Allowed
	YOGHURT	Allowed	Allowed	Allowed
	BUTTER/ GHEE	Allowed	Allowed	Allowed
	CHEESE	Possibly – no rennet	Possibly	Possibly
	CHICKEN	Possibly	Halal – only	Possibly
	MUTTON	Possibly	Halal – only	Possibly
	BEEF	Forbidden	Halal – only	Forbidden
	PORK	Forbidden	Forbidden	Probably not
	FISH	Probably not	Allowed – with fins and scales only	Possibly
	LARD	Forbidden	Forbidden	Forbidden
Some basic guidelines concerning special beliefs and customs affecting the process of menu planning		Will not eat food where the taking of life is involved. Devout Hindus will not eat eggs, meat or fish. The cow is a sacred animal so devout Hindus will not eat beef. Most Hindus rely on beans, pulses, nuts, milk, seeds, yoghurt and white cheese for protein. The staple cereals are wheat, made into chapattis, and rice. Some Hindus may refuse food if the ingredients are unknown or if cooking vessels have not been kept separate.	Halal meat is eaten as well as Kosher meals provided for the Jewish religion. Animal fat should be Halal. Devout Muslims prefer separate utensils to be used for preparing and serving food. Many products will be refused until the purity of the ingredients is known. Rice and bread are the staple food of most Muslims. All kinds of alcohol are prohibited. Water is used at meals.	Some Sikhs are vegetarians, others may eat chicken, lamb and fish. Most Sikhs take no alcohol. It is unusual for beef and pork to be eaten.
Points to consider (a) Separate set of cooking utensils and cutlery should be available to respect religious/spiritual requirements. (b) Under no circumstances should utensils be mixed when preparing or serving food for Muslim patients – especially with pork. (c) Please refer to resource pack for further information.		A number of festivals exist which may involve fasting. The dates of the festivals vary as do the times of fasting. Birthdays of: – Lord Shiva – Mahashivratri – Lord Rama – Rama Navami – Lord Krishna – Janamashtami. Some Hindus will eat pork. Some Hindus fast one or two days a week from dawn to dusk. Devout Hindus will not eat onions or garlic.	There are two major festivals each year. The Festival of Eid-ul-Fitr marks the end of the month of fasting (Ramadan). The Festival of Eid-ul-Adha falls on the day after Hajj. Pregnant Muslim women are not required to fast during Ramadan unless they wish to. Ramadan's 40 days of fasting means abstaining from all food, drink, smoking and marital relations during daylight hours.	Some devout Sikhs fast once or twice a week from dawn to dusk. Main festivals: – New Year – Baisakhi – Festival of Lights – Divali – Birth of Guru Nanak

	UNITS	JUDAISM	VEGETARIANISM	VEGANISM
Specific cultural and religious requirements to be considered in the process of menu planning	EGGS MILK YOGHURT BUTTER/ GHEE CHEESE CHICKEN MUTTON BEEF PORK FISH LARD	Allowed – Dairy products must be kept apart from meat products in cooking and eating Kosher only Kosher only Kosher only Forbidden Allowed – with fins and scales only Forbidden	Allowed Allowed Allowed – no gelatine Allowed Allowed – no rennet Forbidden Forbidden Forbidden Forbidden Forbidden Forbidden	Forbidden Forbidden Forbidden Forbidden Forbidden Forbidden Forbidden Forbidden Forbidden Forbidden Forbidden
Some basic guidelines concerning special beliefs and customs affecting the process of menu planning		Orthodox Jews keep meat and dairy food apart during cooking and eating. Shellfish are forbidden. Herbivorous birds are permitted, e.g. duck goose, turkey. Birds of prey may not be eaten. All animals and birds eaten must be koshered. Only the meat of animals with a cloven hoof and those that chew the cud are eaten, e.g. sheep, ox, goat, deer.	Demi-vegetarians exclude red meat but eats white poultry and fish. Lacto-vegetarians eat milk and cheese but not eggs, fish, meat or products produced by taking life. Lacto-ovo-vegetarians eat milk, cheese and eggs. Yoghurt should not be eaten if it contains gelatine and hard cheese should be made with non-animal rennet. Meat and fish are replaced by beans, pulses, nuts, seeds, cereals, mushrooms and quorn.	Vegans go further than vegetarians as they exclude all animal products including honey. Essential nutrients can be obtained from cereals, beans, pulses, nuts, seeds, fruits and vegetables and fungi. Manufactured products using soya and beans (e.g. tofu, soya milk) and microprotein (e.g. quorn) add extra protein to the diet.
Points to consider (a) Separate set of cooking utensils and cutlery should be available to respect religious/spiritual requirements. (b) Under no circumstances should utensils be mixed when preparing or serving food for Muslim patients – especially with pork. (c) Please refer to resource pack for further information.		Various festivals exist when traditional foods are eaten. Fasts last all day and night. Main festivals: – New Year – Rosh Hashana – Fast Day – Yom Kippur – Feast of Tabernacles – Sukkot – Dairy Festival – Pentecost The Sabbath lasts from dusk on Friday till nightfall on Saturday.	Strictly a vegetarian is defined as one whose diet does not include flesh, fish or fowl. (However, variations exist according to the individual reasons for eating a vegetarian diet.) Many margarines contain animal products and are unsuitable.	Many margarines contain animal products and are unsuitable. Specific pure margarines are available. Lemon and herb teas are preferred. Yeast extracts add essential B vitamins to the diet.

Source: Tony Lingiah on behalf of Race and Culture Project Group 1997

APPENDIX 4
Personal Care

Standard Reference No: RCAR3

Hospital Reference No: 3

Topic: Race & Culture

Sub Topic: Personal Care

Care Group: All patients from
minority groups

Hospital Service Standard

Implement Standard by:
1998/99

Audit Standard by: 1998/99

Signature of Chief Executive:

Initiated by: The Race & Culture
Group

Standard Statement		
Broadmoor Hospital Authority is committed to ensuring the provision of appropriate personal care, which is sensitive to the specific requirements of all patients from ethnic minority groups.		
Structure	Process	Outcome
1. Awareness training for all disciplines. 2. Systems are in place to access skin, hair and beauty products. 3. Assessment of need is available. 4. Current information with regard to beauty products is available.	1. Staff are sensitive and aware of specific patient requirements via assessment of need, which include: – appropriate skin and hair care – availability of specific beauty products – personal cleanliness/hygiene issues for specific groups – appropriateness of gender of care worker in the delivery of personal care/intimate requirements. 2. If products are required, these are placed on requisition and processed via the Patients' Cash Office.	1. Patients are provided with specific requirements appropriate to their personal care and hygiene. 2. Staff deliver culture-sensitive care within hospital protocols.

AUDIT PROTOCOL

Audit Reference No: RCAR3   **Hospital Service Standard**

Hospital Reference No: 3

Audit objective: That there is appropriate provision of personal care, which is specific to the requirements of all patients from ethnic minority groups?

Time frame: Initial audit to be completed within six months, thereafter on an annual basis.

Sample: All wards which are identified by the resident population of ethnic minority patients.

Auditors: Members of the Race & Culture Group   **Date:** 1998/99

Target group	Method	Code	Audit criteria
Staff	Ask	S1 P1 O2	Is awareness training provided for all disciplines?
Staff	Ask	S1	Are staff aware of the procedure of obtaining beauty products for patients who require them?
Nursing process/ treatment plan	Chart audit	S3 P1	Is an assessment of need completed for all patients?
Noticeboards/ information folders	Observe	S4	Is current and up-to-date information available on the type of products that patients may require?
Staff	Ask	P1	Are staff sensitive and aware of specific requirements of patients from ethnic minority groups?
Patients	Ask	O1	Are patients provided with specific requirements appropriate to their personal care and hygiene?
Staff	Ask		

APPENDIX 5
Religious and spiritual needs

Standard Reference No: RCAR4

Hospital Reference No: 4

Topic: Race & Culture

Sub Topic: Religious & Spiritual Needs

Care Group: All patients

Hospital Service Standard

Implement Standard by: 1998/99

Audit Standard by: 1998/99

Signature of Chief Executive:

Initiated by: The Race & Culture Group

Standard Statement		
Broadmoor Hospital Authority observes the religious and spiritual beliefs of all patients.		
Structure	**Process**	**Outcome**
1. Relevant information is provided on all wards about religious facilities available.	1. Information regarding the patients' religious/spiritual needs are to be identified on the information sheet contained within the nursing process/case notes.	1. All patients have access to facilities which observe their religious/spiritual beliefs.
2. All necessary facilities are made available to enable patients to fulfil their religious/spiritual needs.	2. A thorough nursing assessment of religious/spiritual needs is completed and recorded in the nursing process documentation.	
3. All wards have been supplied with a resource pack re: information about different religious groups, e.g. staff to observe ablution requirements for Muslim prayer, respect fasting requirements for Muslim prayer during Ramadan.	3. A referral to the Hospital Chaplain is required to access visiting chaplains or spiritual advisers of all other faiths/denominations.	
4. Hospital Chaplain co-ordinates access to visiting chaplains of all faiths/denominations.	4. The ward facilitates access to all necessary religious/spiritual activity/worship, and any intervention or request of a spiritual nature is to be cross-referenced in the 'Record of Chaplaincy intervention'.	

AUDIT PROTOCOL

Audit Reference No: RCAR4   **Hospital Service Standard**

Hospital Reference No: 4

Audit objective: That Broadmoor Hospital Authority observes the religious and spiritual beliefs of all patients.

Timeframe: Initial audit to be completed within six months, thereafter on an annual basis.

Sample: All wards which are identified by the resident population of ethnic minority patients.

Auditors: Members of the Race & Culture Group   **Date:** 1998/99

Target group	Method	Code	Audit criteria
Noticeboards/ information folders	Observe	S1	Is information provided with regard to the religious facilities available to patients?
Information sheet in nursing process/ case notes	Chart audit	P1	Is information regarding the patients' religious/spiritual needs identified on the information sheet contained within the nursing process/case notes?
Nursing process	Chart audit	P2	Has a thorough nursing assessment of religious/spiritual needs been completed?
Information available at ward level	Observe	S3	Is a resource pack available to staff re: information about different religious groups?
Nursing process	Chart audit	S3 O1	Is a referral made to the Hospital Chaplain should access be required to visiting chaplains or spiritual advisors of all other faiths/denominations?
Staff	Ask		
Patients	Ask	O1	Are all patients provided with access to facilities which observe their religious/spiritual beliefs?
Staff	Ask		

References

Aakster, C.W. (1986) 'Concepts in alternative medicine.' *Social Science and Medicine 22*, 265–273.

Aboud, T.E. (1987) 'The development of ethnic self-identification and attitudes.' In J.S. Pinney and M.J. Rotherans (eds) *Children's Ethnic Socialization: Pluralism and Development*. Newbury Page, CA: Sage.

Adebimpe, V.R. (1984) 'American blacks and psychiatry.' *Transcultural Psychiatric Research Review 21*, 83–111.

Adebimpe, V.R. (1994) 'Race, racism, and epidemiological surveys.' *Hospital and Community Psychiatry 45*, 27–31.

Agbolegbe, R. (1984) 'Fighting the racist disease.' *Nursing Times 80*, 16, 18–20.

Akinsanya, J. (1988) 'Ethnic minority nurses, midwives and health visitors: what role for them in the NHS?' *New Community 14*, 444–450.

Alexander, Z. and Dewgee, A. (1984) *Wonderful Adventures of Mrs Seacole in Many Lands*. Bristol: Falling Wall Press.

Al-Issa, I. (1995) 'The illusion of reality or the reality of illusion.' *British Journal of Psychiatry 166*, 3, 368–373.

Allen, J.J., Rack, P.H. and Vaddadi, K.S. (1977) 'Differences in the effects of clomipramine on English and Asian volunteers. Preliminary report on a pilot study.' *Postgraduate Medical Journal 53*, 79–86.

Allport, W. (1979) *The Nature of Prejudice*. Reading, MA: Addison-Wesley.

Aspinall, P.J. (1995) 'Department of Health's requirements for mandatory collection of data on ethnic groups of inpatients.' *British Medical Journal 311*, 1006–1009.

Balarajan, R. and Raleigh, V.S. (1992) 'The ethnic populations of England and Wales: the 1991 Census.' *Health Trends 24*, 113–116.

Balarajan, R. and Raleigh, V.S. (1993b) *Ethnicity in Health: A Guide for the NHS*. London: Department of Health.

Balarajan, R. and Raleigh, V.S. (1993a) *The Health of the Nation: Ethnicity and Health*. London: Department of Health.

Bartlett, A. (1997) 'Transcultural issues in forensic psychiatry.' *Current Medical Literature*.

Bateson, G. (1973) *Steps to an Ecology of Mind*. Frogmore: Paladin.

Bean, R.B. (1906) 'Some racial peculiarities of the Negro brain.' *American Journal of Anatomy 5*, 353–415.

Bebbington, P.E., Feeney, S.T., Flannigan, C.B., Glover, G.R., Lewis, S.W. and Wing, J.K. (1994) 'Inner London collaborative audit of admissions in two health districts.' II: Ethnicity and the use of the Mental Health Act. *British Journal of Psychiatry 165*, 743–749.

Bebbington, P.E., Hurry, J. and Tennant, C. (1981) 'Psychiatric disorders in selected immigrant groups in Camberwell.' *Social Psychiatry 16*, 43–51.

Begue, J.-M. (1996) 'French Psychiatry in Algeria 1830–1962: from colonial to transcultural.' *History of Psychiatry vii*, 533–548.

Beishon S., Virdee, S. and Hazell, A. (1995) *Nursing in a Multi-Ethnic NHS.* London: Policy Studies Institute.

Beliappa, J. (1991) *Illness or Distress, Alternative Model of Mental Health.* London: Confederation of Indian Organisations.

Bell, C. (1993) *Ritual Theory, Ritual Practice.* New York: Oxford University Press.

Berkshire Health Commission (1995) *Handbook on Ethnic Minority Issues: A Guide for GPs and Practice Staff on the Care of Individual Patients.* Berkshire: Berkshire Health Commission.

Bhatt, A., Tomenson, B. and Benjamin, S. (1989) 'Transcultural patterns of somatization in primary care: a preliminary report.' *Journal of Psychosomatic Research 33*, 671–680.

Bhopal, R., (1997) 'Is research into ethnicity and health racist, unsound or important science?' *British Medical Journal 314*, 1751–1756.

Bhugra, D. (1997) 'Setting up psychiatric services: Cross-cultural issues in planning and delivery.' International Journal of Social Psychiatry 43, 16–28.

Bhugra, D., Desai, M. and Baldwin, D.S. (1999) 'Attempted suicide in West London. Incidence rates across ethnic communities.' *Psychological Medicine 29*, 1125–1130.

Bhugra, D., Hilwig, M., Hossein, B., Marceau, H., Neehall, J., Leff, J., Mallett, R. and Der, G. (1996) 'First contact incidence rates of schizophrenia in Trinidad and one-year follow-up.' *British Journal of Psychiatry 169*, 587–592.

Bhugra, D., Leff, J., Mallett, R., Der, G., Corridan, B. and Rudge, S. (1997) 'Incidence and outcome of schizophrenia in whites, African-Caribbeans and Asians in London.' *Psychological Medicine 27*, 791–798.

Bhui, K. and Bhugra, D. (1997) 'Cross-cultural competencies in the psychiatric assessment.' *British Journal of Hospital Medicine 57*, 492–496.

Bhui, K., Brown, P., Hardie, T., Watson, J.P. and Parrott, J. (1998a) 'African-Caribbean men remanded to Brixton Prison.' *British Journal of Psychiatry 172*, 337–344.

Bhui, K., Brown, P., Hardie, T., Watson, J.P. and Parrott, J. (1998b) 'Psychiatric and forensic characteristics and outcome of final court appearance.' *British Journal of Psychiatry 172*, April.

Bhui, K. and Carrs, S. (1997) *Psychiatric Service Provision for African and Caribbean Populations.* Needs Assessment Factsheet 10, The Sainsbury Centre for Mental Health.

Bhui, K., Strathdee, G. and Sufraz, R. (1993) 'Asian inpatients in a district psychiatric unit: an examination of presenting features and routes into care.' *International Journal of Social Psychiatry 39*, 208–220.

Birchwood, M., Cochrane, R., Macmillan, F., Copestake, S., Kucharska, J. and Carriss, M. (1992) 'The influence of ethnicity and family structure on relapse in first-episode schizophrenia.' *British Journal of Psychiatry 161*, 783–790.

Blom-Cooper, L., Browne, M., Dolan, R. and Murphy, E. (1992) *Report of the Committee of Inquiry into Complaints about Ashworth Hospital.* London: HMSO.

Boast, N. and Chesterman, P. (1995) 'Black people in secure psychiatric facility; patterns of processing and the role of stereotypes.' *British Journal of Criminology 35,* 2.

Boateng, P. (1997) Quoted in *Health Service Journal,* 12.9.97.

Bolton, P. (1984) 'Management of Compulsory Admitted Patients to a High Security Unit.' *International Journal of Social Psychiatry 30,* 2, 671–684.

Bourne, J., Bridges, L. and Searle, C. (1994) *Outcast England, How Schools Exclude Black Children.* London: Institute of Race Relations.

Bowker, J. (1983) *Worlds of Faith: Religious Belief and Practice in Britain Today.* London: Ariel Books.

Bowker, J. (1987) *Licensed Insanities: Religions and Belief in God in the Contemporary World.* London: Dartman, Longman and Todd.

Bowker, J. (ed) (1997) *The Oxford Dictionary of World Religions.* Oxford and New York: Oxford University Press.

Bowl, R. and Barnes, M. (1990) 'Race, racism and mental health social work: implications for Local Authority policy and training.' *Research, Policy and Planning 8,* 12–18.

Bracken, P.J., Greenslade, L., Griffin, B. and Smyth, M. (1998) 'Mental health and ethnicity: an Irish dimension.' *British Journal of Psychiatry 172,* February, 103–106.

Brandon, D. (1991) *Innovation Without Change? Consumer Power in Psychiatric Services.* London: Macmillan.

Brewin, C. (1980) 'Explaining the lower rates of psychiatric treatment among Asian immigrants to the United Kingdom: a preliminary study.' *Social Psychiatry 15,* 17–19.

Brindle, D. (1997) 'Young blacks "in fear" of mental health services.' *Guardian,* 8 September, p.2.

Broadmoor Hospital (1998a) *Standards for Women's Services.* Berkshire: Broadmoor Hospital Authority.

Broadmoor Hospital (1998b) *A Charter for You.* Berkshire: Broadmoor Hospital Authority.

Brown, R.P. and Kocsis, J.H. (1984) 'Sudden death and antipsychotic drugs.' *Hospital and Community Psychiatry 35,* 486–491.

Browne, D. (1990) *Black People, Mental Health and the Courts: An Exploratory Study into the Psychiatric process as it Affects Black Defendants at Magistrates Courts.* London: NACRO.

Browne, D. (1995) 'The black experience of mental health law.' *Mental Health Matters: A Reader.* Milton Keynes: Open University.

Buchanan, A. (1998) 'Treatment compliance in schizophrenia.' *Advances in Psychiatric Treatment 4,* 4, 227–234.

Bullard, H. and Bond, M. (1988) 'Secure Units: why they are needed.' *Medicine, Science and the Law 28,* 4, 312–318.

Burke, A.W. (1974) 'First admissions and planning in Jamaica.' *Social Psychiatry 9,* 39–45.

Burke, A.W. (1976a) 'Socio-cultural determinants of attempted suicide among West Indians in Birmingham: ethnic origin and immigrant status.' *British Journal of Psychiatry 129,* 261–266.

Burke, A.W. (1976b) 'Attempted suicide among Asian immigrants in Birmingham.' *British Journal of Psychiatry 128,* 528–533.

Burke, A.W. (1984) 'Racism and psychological disturbance among West Indians in Britain.' *International Journal of Social Psychiatry 30,* 50–68.

Burleigh, M (1997) *Ethics and Extermination: Reflections on Nazi Genocide.* Cambridge. Cambridge University Press.

Callan, A.F. (1996) 'Schizophrenia in Afro-Caribbean immigrants.' *Journal of the Royal Society of Medicine 89,* 253–256.

Campling, P. (1989) 'Race, culture and psychotherapy.' *Psychiatric Bulletin 13,* 550–551.

Carothers, J.C. (1953) *The African Mind in Health and Disease. A Study in Ethnopsychiatry. WHO Monograph Series No. 17.* Geneva: World Health Organisation.

Carpenter, L. and Brockington, I.F. (1980) 'A study of mental illness in Asians, West Indians and Africans living in Manchester.' *British Journal of Psychiatry 137,* 201–205.

Carr, J.E. and Vitaliano, P.P. (1985) 'The theoretical implications of converging research on depression and the culture-bound syndromes.' In A. Kleinman and Byron Good (eds) *Culture and Depression.*

Cartwright, S.A. (1851) 'Report on the diseases and physical peculiarities of the Negro race.' *New Orleans Medical and Surgical Journal,* May, 691–715. Reprinted in A.C. Caplan, H.T. Engelhardt and J.J. McCartney (eds) *Concepts of Health and Disease.* Massachusetts: Addison-Wesley.

Castro-Caldas, A., Petersson, K.M., Reis, A., Stone-Elander, S. and Ingvar, M. (1998) 'The illiterate brain: learning to read and write during childhood influences the functional organisation of the adult brain.' *Brain 121,* 1053–1063.

Chen, E., Harrison, G. and Standen, P. (1991) 'Management of first episode psychiatric illness in AfroCaribbeans.' *British Journal of Psychiatry 158,* 517–522.

Chiswick, D. (1992) 'Compulsory treatment of patients with psychopathic disorder: an abnormally aggressive and seriously irresponsible exercise?' *Criminal Behaviour and Mental Health 2,* 106–113.

Clifford, J. (1988) *The Predicament of Culture: Twentieth-Century Ethnography, Literature and Art.* Cambridge, MA: Harvard University Press.

Cobb, W.M. (1942) 'Physical anthropology of the American Negro.' *American Journal of Physical Anthropology 29,* 113–223.

Cochrane, R. (1977) 'Mental illness in immigrants to England and Wales: an analysis of mental hospital admissions, 1971.' *Social Psychiatry 12,* 25–35.

Cochrane, R. and Bal, S.S. (1987) 'Migration and schizophrenia: an examination of five hypotheses.' *Social Psychiatry 22,* 181–191.

Cochrane, R. and Bal, S.S. (1989) 'Mental hospital admission rates of immigrants to England: a comparison of 1971 and 1981.' *Social Psychiatry and Psychiatric Epidemiology 24*, 2–11.

Cochrane, R. and Stopes-Roe, M. (1977) 'Psychological and social adjustment of Asian immigrants to Britain: a community survey.' *Social Psychiatry 12*, 195–206.

Cochrane, R. and Stopes-Roe, M. (1981) 'Psychological symptom levels in Indian immigrants to England – a comparison with native English.' *Psychological Medicine 11*, 319–327.

Coid, J.W. (1992) 'DSM-III diagnosis in criminal psychopaths: a way forward.' *Criminal Behaviour and Mental Health 2*, 78–93.

Coldwell, J.B. and Naismith, L.J. (1989) 'Violent incidents on special care wards in a Special Hospital.' *Medicine, Science and the Law 29*, 2, 116–123.

Cole, E., Leavey, G., King, M., Johnson-Sabine, E. and Hoar, A. (1995) 'Pathways to care for patients with a first episode of psychosis. A comparison of ethnic groups.' *British Journal of Psychiatry 167*, 770–776.

Comer, J.P. (1985) 'Black violence and public policy.' In L. Curtis (ed) *American Violence and Public Policy*. New Haven: Yale University Press.

Commander, M.J., Sashidharan, S.P., Odell, S.M. and Surtees, P.G. (1997) 'Access to mental health care in an inner-city health district. I: Pathways into and within specialist psychiatric services. II: Association with demographic factors.' *British Journal of Psychiatry 170*, 312–320.

Commission for Racial Equality (1989a) *The Experience of Health and Mental Health in an Ethnic Minority Group*. London: Commission for Racial Equality.

Commission for Racial Equality (1989b) *Training: The Implementation of Equal Opportunities at Work in Policy and Planning*. Vol. V. London: Commission for Racial Equality.

Commission for Racial Equality (1995a) Unpublished joint study, with Mental Health Act Commission, on civil detentions under the Mental Health Act.

Commission for Racial Equality (1995b) *Position Paper, The Race Implications of the Mental (Patients in the Community) Health Bill*. London: Commission for Racial Equality.

Commission for Racial Equality (1997) *Exclusion from School and Racial Equality*. London: Commission for Racial Equality.

Cooper, J.E., Kendell, R.E., Gurland, B.J., Sharpe, L., Copeland, J.R.M. and Simon, R. (1972) *Psychiatric Diagnosis in New York and London. Maudsley Monograph No 20*. Oxford: Oxford University Press.

Cope, R. (1989) 'The compulsory detention of Afro-Caribbeans under the Mental Health Act.' *New Community 15*, 3, 343–353.

Cope, R. and Ndegwa, D. (1990) 'Ethnic differences in admission to a regional secure unit.' *Journal of Forensic Psychiatry 3*, 365–378.

Cowie, G. (1992) 'Learning from Our Experiences.' *Let's Talk Entre Nous 17*, 5, May 4–5.

Crowley, J.J. and Simmons, S. (1992) 'Mental health, race and ethnicity: a retrospective study of the care of ethnic minorities and whites in a psychiatric unit.' *Journal of Advanced Nursing 17*, 1078–1087.

D'Aquili, E.G., Laughlin, C. and McManus, J. (eds) (1990) *Brain, Symbol, and Experience: Toward a Neurohenomenology of Human Consciousness.* Boston: New Science Library.

Davies, S., Thornicroft, G., Leese, M., Higgingbotham, A. and Phelan, M. (1996) 'Ethnic differences in risk of compulsory psychiatric admission among representative cases of psychosis in London.' *British Medical Journal 312*, 533–537.

Davis, J.M. and Zhang, M.Y. (1988) 'Sudden death in psychiatric patients.' *Psychiatric Annals 18*, 311–319.

Dean, G., Downing, H. and Shelley, E. (1981) 'First admissions of native-born and immigrants to psychiatric hospitals in south-east England 1976.' *British Journal of Psychiatry 139*, 506–512.

Deeley, P.Q. (1999) 'Medicine, psychiatry, and the ecology of mind' (in press in *Medicine and Anthropology*)

Deeley, P.Q. (1999) 'Ecological understandings of mental and physical illness.' *Philosophy, Psychiatry and Psychology 6*, 2.

Department of Health (1990) *Caring for People: Community Care in the Next Decade and Beyond.* London: Department of Health Policy and Practice Guidance.

Department of Health (1992) *Report of the Committee of Inquiry into Complaints about Ashworth Hospital.* Vols 1 and 2. Cm-2028–1 and 2028–11. London: HMSO.

Department of Health (1995) Building Bridges – A guide to the arrangements for inter-agency working for care and protection of severely mentally ill people. London: Department of Health.

Department of Health (1996a) *NHS Complaints Procedure.* London: Department of Health.

Department of Health (1996b) *NHS Patients Charter.* London: Department of Health.

Department of Health (1997a) *NHS Mental Health Services Charter.* London: Department of Health.

Department of Health (1997b) *The New NHS: Modern and Dependable.* London: Department of Health.

Department of Health (1998a) *NHS Hospital and Community Health Services Non-Medical Staff in England: 1987–1997.* Bulletin 1998/15, May. London: Government Statistical Service.

Department of Health (1998b) *Hospital, Public Health Medicine and Community Health Service Medical and Dental Staff in England 1987 to 1997.* Bulletin 1998/27, August London: Government Statistical Service.

Department of Health (1998c) *Patients Formally Detained in Hospitals under the Mental Health Act 1983 and Other Legislation.* London: Government Statistical Services.

Department of Health and Home Office (1992a) *Services for people from black and ethnic minority groups: issues of race and culture.* Vol 6 of *Review of Health and Social Services for Mentally Disordered Offenders and Others Requiring Similar Services.* London: HMSO.

Department of Health and Home Office (1992b) *The Care Programme Approach. Services for People from Black and Ethnic Minority Groups. Issues of Race and Culture – A discussion paper.* HS(90) 23/LAS(90)(11). London: HMSO.

Department of Health and Home Office (1993) *Review of Health and Social Services for Mentally Disordered Offenders and Others Requiring Similar Services: Special Issues and Differing Needs* Vol. 5. (Chairman: Reed) London: HMSO.

Department of Health and Social Security (1980) *Report of the Committee of Inquiry into Rampton Hospital.* Cmnd 8073. London: HMSO.

Department of Health/NHS Executive High Secure Psychiatric Services Commissioning Board (1997) *A Consultation Event: The Future Provision of Secure Psychiatric Services for Black People.* London: Department of Health.

Diaz, R. (1998) Ethnicity and Housing. London: Shelter.

Dohrenwend, B.P., Levav, I., Shrout, P.E., Schwartz, S., Naveh, G., Link, B.G., Skodol, A.E. and Stueve, A. (1992) 'Socio-economic status and psychiatric disorders: the causation-selection issue.' *Science 255*, 946–952.

Down, J.L.M. (1866) 'Observations on an ethnic classification of idiots.' *Lectures and Reports from the London Hospital for 1866.* Reprinted in C. Thompson (ed) *The Origins of Modern Psychiatry.* Chichester: Wiley. pp.15–18.

Drever, F. and Whitehead, M. (eds) (1997) *Health Inequalities.* London: HMSO.

Dunn, J. and Fahy, T.A. (1990) 'Police admissions to a psychiatric hospital: demographic and clinical differences between ethnic groups.' *British Journal of Psychiatry 156*, 373–378.

Eagles, J.M. (1991) 'The relationship between schizophrenia and immigration. Are there alternatives to psychosocial hypotheses?' *British Journal of Psychiatry 159*, 783–789.

Eagles, J.M. (1992) 'Are polio viruses a cause of schizophrenia?' *British Journal of Psychiatry 160*, 598–600.

Esmail, A. and Everington, S. (1993) 'Racial discrimination against doctors from ethnic minorities.' *British Medical Journal 306*, 691–692.

Esmail, A. and Everington, S. (1994) 'General Medical Council complaints may reflect racism.' *British Medical Journal 308*, 1374.

Esmail, A. and Everington, S. (1997) 'Asian doctors are still being discriminated against.' *British Medical Journal 314*, 1619.

Esmail, A., Everington, S. and Doyle, H. (1998) 'Racial discrimination in the allocation of distinction awards.' *British Medical Journal, 316*, 193–195.

Esmail, A., Nelson, P., Primarolo, D. and Toma, T. (1995) 'Acceptance into medical school and racial discrimination.' *British Medical Journal 310*, 25 Febuary, 501–502.

Eysenck, H.J. (1971) *Race, Intelligence and Education.* London: Temple Smith.

Farnham, F.R. and Kennedy. H.G. (1997) 'Acute excited states and sudden death.' *British Medical Journal 315*, 1107–1108.

Fernando, S. (1988) *Race and Culture in Psychiatry.* London: Billing and Sons Ltd.

Fernando, S. (1991) *Mental Health, Race and Culture.* Basingstoke and London: Macmillan in association with MIND.

Fernando, S. (1996) 'Black people working in white institutions: lessons from personal experience.' *The Journal of Systemic Consultation and Management,* 7.

Fernando, S. (1998) 'Grasping the nettle.' *Open Mind 91,* May/June, 15.

Fernando, S., Ndegwa, D. and Wilson, M. (1998) *Forensic Psychiatry, Race and Culture.* London: Routledge.

Fitzgerald, M. (1993) *Ethnic Minorities and the Criminal Justice System.* Research Study No.20 for the Royal Commission on Criminal Justice. London: HMSO.

Fitzgerald, M. and Sibbitt, R. (1997) *Ethnic Monitoring in Police Forces: A Beginning.* Home Office Research Study 173. London: Home Office.

Flaskerud, J.H. and Hu, L.T. (1992a) 'Relationship of ethnicity to psychiatric diagnosis.' *Journal of Nervous Mental Disorders 180,* 296–303.

Flaskerud, J.H. and Hu, L. (1992b) 'Racial/ethnic identity and amount and type of psychiatric treatment.' *American Journal of Psychiatry 149,* 379–384.

Forshaw, D. and Rollin, H. (1990) 'The history of law and psychiatry in Europe.' In R. Bluglass and P. Bowden (eds) *Principles and Practice of Forensic Psychiatry.* London: Churchill Livingstone.

Fortes, M. (1966) 'Religious premises and logical techniques in divinatory ritual.' In J. Huxley (ed) *A Discussion of Ritualisation of Behaviours in Animals and Men.* Philosophical Transactions of the Royal Society of London, Series B, vol. 251 Biological Sciences. London: Royal Society.

Foucault, M. (1988) *Politics Philosophy Culture. Interviews and Other writings 1977–1984* (ed. L.D. Kritzman). London: Routledge.

Francis, E., David, J., Johnson and Sashidhasan, S.P. (1989) 'Black people and psychiatry in the United Kingdom. An alternative to institutional care.' *Psychiatric Bulletin 13,* 482–485.

Freud, S. (1907) 'Obsessive actions and religious practices.' In J. Strachey *et al.* (editors and translators) *The Standard Edition of the Complete Psychological Works of Sigmund Freud,* 24 vols, 1953–1974. Vol.9 (1959), 115–27. London: Hogarth Press.

Friston, K. and Frith, C. (1995) 'Schizophrenia: a disconnection syndrome?' *Clinical Neuroscience 3,* 89–97.

Fryer, P. (1993) *Aspects of British Black History.* London: Index Books.

Furnham, A. and Shiekh, S. (1993) 'Gender, generational and social support correlates of mental health in Asian immigrants.' *International Journal of Social Psychiatry 39,* 22–33.

Gamwell, L. and Tomes, N. (1995) *Madness in America: Cultural and Medical Perceptions of Mental Illness Before 1914.* New York: Cornell University Press.

Gay, V. (1978) 'Reductionism and redundancy in the analysis of religious forms.' *Zygon 13,* 2, 169–183.

Geertz, C. (1973) *The Interpretation of Cultures.* New York, NY: Basic Books.

Geertz, C. (1985) 'From the native's point of view: on the nature of anthropological understanding.' In R. Shweder and R. LeVine (eds) *Culture Theory: Essays on Mind, Self, and Emotion.* Cambridge: Cambridge University Press.

Gelder, M., Gath, D. and Mayou, R. (1989) *Oxford Textbook of Psychiatry*. Oxford: Oxford University Press.

Gillam, S.J., Jarman, B., White, P. and Law, R. (1989) 'Ethnic differences in consultation rates in urban general practice.' *British Medical Journal 299*, 953–957.

Glover, G.R. (1989) 'The pattern of psychiatric admissions of Caribbean-born immigrants in London.' *Social Psychiatry and Psychiatric Epidemiology 24*, 49–56.

Glover, G.R. (1991) 'The use of inpatient psychiatric care by immigrants in a London borough.' *International Journal of Social Psychiatry 37*, 121–134.

Glover, G.R., Flannigan, C.B., Feeney, S.T., Wing, J.K., Bebbington, P.E. and Lewis, S.W. (1994) 'Admission of British Caribbeans to mental hospitals: is it a cohort effect?' *Social Psychiatry and Psychiatric Epidemiology 29*, 282–284.

Glover, G. and Malcolm, G. (1988) 'The prevalence of depot neuroleptic treatment among West Indians and Asians in the London borough of Newham.' *Social Psychiatry and Psychiatric Epidemiology 23*, 281–284.

Goater, N. et al. (1999) 'Ethnicity and outcome of psychosis.' *British Journal of Psychiatry, 175* 34–42.

Goffman, E. (1968) *Asylums*. Harmondsworth: Penguin.

Good, B. (1995) *Medicine, Rationality, and Experience*. Cambridge: Cambridge University Press.

Gordon, H. (1996) 'Psychopaths in special hospitals.' *British Journal of Psychiatry 168*, (letter), 653.

Gostin, L. (1986) *Institutions Observed: Towards a New Concept of Secure Provision in Mental Health*. London: King's Fund.

Gottesman, I.I. (1991) Schizophrenia Genesis: The Origins of Madness. New York, NY: Freeman.

Government Statistical Service (1998) *Civil Service Statistics 1997*. London: Government Statistical Service.

Gowers, S., Entwistle, K., Cooke, N., Okpalugo, B. and Kenyon, A. (1993) 'Social and family factors in adolescent psychiatry.' *Journal of Adolescence 16*, 353–366.

Green, E.M. (1914) 'Psychoses among Negroes – a comparative study.' *Journal of Nervous and Mental Disorder 41*, 697–708.

Greenwood, A. (1995) *Mental Illness and Those Who are Ethnically Distinctive*. Bradford: Lynfield Mount Hospital.

Grounds, A.T. (1987) 'Detention of "psychopathic disorder" patients in Special Hospital: critical issues.' *British Journal of Psychiatry 151*, 474–478.

Gunn, J. (1992) 'Personality disorders and forensic psychiatry.' *Criminal Behaviour and Mental Health 2*, 2, 202–211.

Gunn, J., Maden, T. and Swinton, M. (1991) *Mentally Disorders Prisoners*. London: Home Office

Gupta, S. (1991) 'Psychosis in migrants from the Indian subcontinent and English-born controls. A preliminary study on the use of psychiatric services.' *British Journal of Psychiatry 159*, 222–225.

Gupta, S. (1992) 'Psychosis in Asian immigrants from the Indian subcontinent: preliminary findings from a follow-up study including a survey of general practitioners.' *Social Psychiatry and Psychiatric Epidemiology* 27, 242–244.

Gupta, S. (1993) 'Can environmental factors explain the epidemiology of schizophrenia in immigrant groups?' *Social Psychiatry and Psychiatric Epidemiology* 28, 263–266.

Hall, G.S. (1904) *Adolescence: Its Psychology and Its Relations to Physiology, Anthropology, Sociology, Sex, Crime, Religion and Education.* Vol. II. New York: Appleton D.

Hamilton, J. (1987) 'The management of psychopathic offenders.' *British Journal of Hospital Medicine* 38, 3, 245–250.

Hanauske-Abel, H.M. (1996) 'Not a slippery slope or sudden subversion: German medicine and National Socialism in 1933.' *British Medical Journal 313,* 1453–1463.

Harris, E.C. and Barraclough, B. (1998) 'Excess mortality of mental disorder.' *British Journal of Psychiatry 173,* 11–53.

Harrison, G., Glazebrook, C., Brewin, J., Cantwell, R., Dalkin, T., Fox, R., Jones, P. and Medley, I. (1997) 'Increased incidence of psychotic disorders in migrants from the Caribbean to the United Kingdom.' *Psychological Medicine 27,* 799–806.

Harrison, G., Holton, A., Neilson, D., Owens, D., Boot, D. and Cooper, J. (1989) 'Severe mental disorder in Afro-Caribbean patients: some social, demographic and service factors.' *Psychological Medicine 19,* 683–696.

Harrison G., Owens D., Holton A., Neilson D. and Boot D. (1988) 'A prospective study of severe mental disorder in AfroCaribbean patients.' *Psychological Medicine 18,* 643– 657.

Harvey, I., Williams, M., McGuffin, P. and Toone, B.K. (1990) 'The functional psychoses in Afro-Caribbeans.' *British Journal of Psychiatry 157,* 515–522.

Health Education Authority (1994) *Black and Minority Ethnic Groups in England: Health and Lifestyles.* London: Health Education Authority.

Health Education Authority (1998a) *Mental Health Promotion and Irish People.* London: Health Education Authority.

Health Education Authority (1998b) *Mental Health Promotion and African-Caribbean People.* London: Health Education Authority.

Hemsi, L.K. (1967) 'Psychiatric morbidity of West Indian immigrants: a study of first admissions in London.' *Social Psychiatry 2,* 95–100.

Hicks, C. (1982) 'Racism in Nursing.' *Nursing Times* 5 April.

Hickling, F.W. (1991) 'Psychiatric hospital admission rates in Jamaica 1971 and 1988.' *British Journal of Psychiatry 159,* 817–82.

Hickling, F.W. and Rodgers-Johnson, P. (1995) 'The incidence of first contact schizophrenia in Jamaica.' *British Journal of Psychiatry 167,* 193–196.

Hillam, J. and Evans, C. (1996) 'Neuroleptic drug use in psychiatric intensive therapy units: Problems with complying with the consensus statement.' *Psychiatric Bulletin* 20, 82–84.

Hilton, C. (1996) 'Collecting ethnic group data for inpatients: is it useful?' *British Medical Journal 313,* 923–925.

Home Office (1998) *Prison Statistics 1997*. London: HMSO.

Hood, R. (1992) *Race and Sentencing*. Oxford: Clarendon.

Howlett, M. (1998) *Medication, Non-Compliance and Mentally Disordered Offenders: The Role of Non-Compliance in Homicide by People with Mental Illness and Proposals for Future Policy. A Study of Independent Inquiry Reports*. London: Zito Trust.

Hutchinson, G. and Gilvarry, C. (1998) 'Ethnicity and dissatisfaction with mental health services.' *British Journal of Psychiatry 172* (Correspondence), 95–97.

Hutchinson, G. and McKenzie, K. (1995) 'What is an AfroCaribbean? Implications for Psychiatric Research.' *Psychiatric Bulletin 19*, 700–702.

Hutchinson, G., Takei, N., Fahy, T.A., Bhugra, D., Gilvarry, C., Moran, P., Mallett, R., Sham, P., Leff, J. and Murray, R.M. (1996) 'Morbid risk of schizophrenia in first-degree relatives of white and African-Caribbean patients with psychosis.' *British Journal of Psychiatry 169*, 776–780.

Iganski, P., Spong, A., Mason, D. *et al*. (1998) *Recruiting Minority Ethnic Groups into Nursing, Midwifery and Health Visiting*. London: English National Board for Nursing.

Ineichen, B. (1990) 'The mental health of Asians in Britain.' *British Medical Journal 300*, 1669–1670.

Ineichen, B., Harrison, G. and Morgan, H.G. (1984) 'Psychiatric hospital admissions in Bristol: I. Geographical and ethnic factors.' *British Journal of Psychiatry 145*, 600–604.

Irwin, J. and Cressey, D.R. (1962) 'Thieves, Convicts and Inmate Culture.' *Social Problems 10*, 142–155.

Jasper, L. (1998) 'Black deaths in custody: a human rights perspective.' In A. Leibling (ed) *Deaths of Offenders: The Hidden side of Justice*. Winchester: Waterside Press.

Jawed, S.H. (1991) 'A survey of psychiatrically ill Asian children.' *British Journal of Psychiatry 158*, 268–270.

Jenkins, J.H. (1991) 'The 1990 Stirling Award Essay: Anthropology, expressed emotion, and schizophrenia.' *Ethos 19*, 387–431.

Jensen, A.R. (1969) 'How much can we boost IQ and scholastic achievement?' *Harvard Educational Review 39*, 1–123.

Jones, B.E. and Gray, B.A. (1986) 'Problems in diagnosing schizophrenia and affective disorders among blacks.' *Hospital and Community Psychiatry 37*, 61–65.

Jones, T. (1993) *Britain's Ethnic Minorities*. London: Policy Studies Institute.

Jung, C.G. (1930) 'Your Negroid and Indian behaviour.' *Forum 83*, 4, 193–199.

Kakar, S. (1984) *Shamans, Mystics and Doctors. A Psychological Inquiry into India and its Healing Tradition*. London: Unwin Paperbacks.

Kareem, J. and Littlewood, R. (eds) (1992) *Intercultural Therapy: Themes, Interpretations and Practice*. Oxford: Blackwell Scientific Publications.

Kaye, C. (1998) 'Chance and control: politics and management in secure services.' *Criminal Behaviour and Mental Health 8*, 275–287.

Kaye, C. and Franey, A. (eds) (1998) *Managing High Security Psychiatric Care*. London: Jessica Kingsley Publishers.

Keith, M. (1993) 'From punishment to discipline.' In M. Cross and M. Keith (eds) *Racism, The City and The State.* London: Routledge.

King, M., Coker, E., Leavey, G., Hoare, A. and Johnson-Sabine, E. (1994) 'Incidence of psychotic illness in London: comparison of ethnic groups.' *British Medical Journal 309,* 1115–1119.

Kleinman, A. (1988a) *Rethinking Psychiatry: From Cultural Category to Personal Experience.* New York: The Free Press.

Kleinman, A. (1998b) *The Illness Narratives: Suffering, Healing and the Human Condition.* New York, NY: Basic Books.

Knowles, C. (1991) 'Afro-Caribbeans and schizophrenia: how does psychiatry deal with issues of race, culture and ethnicity.' *Journal of Social Policy 20,* 173–190.

Koffman, J., Fulop, N.J., Pashley, D. and Coleman, K. (1997) 'Ethnicity and use of acute psychiatric beds: one-day survey in North and South Thames regions.' *British Journal of Psychiatry 171,* 238–241.

Kraepelin, E. (1904) 'Vergleichende psychiatrie.' *Zentralblatt Nervenheilkunde und Psychiatrie 27,* 433–437.' Translated by H. Marshall in S.R. Hirsch and M. Shepherd (eds) (1974) *Themes and Variations in European Psychiatry.* Bristol: Wright. pp.3–6.

Kraepelin, E. (1921) *Manic-Depressive Insanity and Paranoia.* Translated and edited by R.M. Barclay and G.M. Robertson. Edinburgh: Livingstone.

Krause, I.B. (1989) 'Sinking heart: A Punjabi communication of distress.' *Social Science Medicine 29,* 563–575.

Krause, I.B., Rosser, R.M., Khiani, M.L. and Lotay, N.S. (1990) 'Psychiatric morbidity among Punjabi medical patients in England measured by General Health Questionnaire.' *Psychological Medicine 20,* 711–719.

Kroeber, A.L. and Kluckhohn, C. (1963) *Culture: A Critical Review of Concepts and Definitions.* New York: Vintage Books.

Lambo, A. (1969) 'Traditional African cultures and Western medicine.' In F.N.L. Poynter (ed) *Medicine and Culture.* London: Wellcome Institute of History of Medicine.

Le Var, R.M.H. (1998) 'Improving Educational Preparation for Transcultural Health Care.' *Nurse Education Today 18,* 519–533.

Leach, E. (1976) *Culture and Communication.* Cambridge: Cambridge University Press.

Leavey, G., King, M., Cole, E., Hoar, A. and Johnson-Sabine, E. (1997) 'First onset psychotic illness; patients and relatives satisfaction with services.' *British Journal of Psychiatry 170,* 53–57.

Lee-Cunin, M. (1989) *Daughters of Seacole, A Study of Black Nurses in West Yorkshire.* Batley: West Yorkshire Low Pay Unit.

Leff, J. (1973) 'Culture and the differentiation of emotional states.' *British Journal of Psychiatry 123,* 299–306.

Leff, J., Wig, N.N., Bedi, H., Menon, D.K., Kuipers, L., Korten, A., Ernberg, G., Day, R., Sartorius, N. and Jablensky, A. (1990) 'Relatives' expressed emotion and the course of schizophrenia in Chandigarh: a two year follow-up of a first-contact sample.' *British Journal of Psychiatry 156,* 351–356.

Leight, A., Johnson, G. and Ingram, A. (1998) *Deaths in Police Custody: Learning the Lessons.* London: Police Policy Directorate, Home Office.

Levi-Strauss, C. (1972) 'The sorcerer and his magic.' In C. Levi-Strauss (ed) *Structural Anthropology.* Harmondsworth: Penguin.

Lewis, G., Croft-Jeffreys, C. and David, A. (1990) 'Are British psychiatrists racist?' *British Journal of Psychiatry 157*, 410–415.

Lewis, P., Rack, P.H., Vaddadi, K.S. and Allen, J.J. (1980) 'Ethnic differences in drug response.' *Postgraduate Medical Journal 56*, Supplement 1, 46–49.

Li, P.L., Jones, I. and Richards, J. (1994) 'The collection of general practice data for psychiatric service contracts.' *Journal of Public Health Medicine 16*, 87–92.

Lifton, R.J. (1982) 'Medicalized killing in Auschwitz.' *Psychiatry 45*, 283–297.

Lin, K.M. and Kleinman, A.M. (1988) 'Psychopathology and clinical course of schizophrenia: a cross-cultural perspective.' *Schizophrenia Bulletin 14*, 555–567.

Lin, K.M., Miller, M.H., Poland, R.E., Nuccio, I. and Yamaguchi, M. (1991) 'Ethnicity and family involvement in the treatment of schizophrenic patients.' *Journal of Nervous and Mental Disease 179*, 631–633.

Lindsey, K.P. and Paul, G.L. (1989) 'Involuntary commitments to public mental institutions: issues involving the over-representation of blacks and assessment of relevant functioning.' *Psychological Bulletin 106*, 171–183.

Lipsedge, M. (1993) 'Mental health: access to care for black and ethnic minority people.' In A. Hopkins and V. Bahl (eds) *Access to Health Care for People from Black and Ethnic Minorities.* London: Royal College of Physicians.

Lipsedge, M. (1994) 'Dangerous Stereotypes.' *Journal of Forensic Psychiatry 5*, 1, 14–19.

Littlewood, R. (1992a) 'Towards an intercultural therapy.' In J. Kareem and R. Littlewood (eds) *Intercultural Therapy.* Oxford: Basil Blackwell.

Littlewood, R. (1992b) 'Psychiatric diagnosis and racial bias: empirical and interpretative approaches.' *Social Science Medicine 34*, 141–149.

Littlewood, R. and Cross, S. (1980) 'Ethnic minorities and psychiatric services.' *Sociology of Health and Illness 2*, 194–201.

Littlewood, R. and Lipsedge, M. (1981) 'Some social and phenomenological characteristics of psychotic immigrants.' *Psychological Medicine 11*, 289–302.

Littlewood, R. and Lipsedge, M. (1989) *Aliens and Alienists: Ethnic Minorities and Psychiatry.* London: Unwin-Hyman.

Littlewood, R. (1986) 'Ethnic minorities and the Mental Health Act.' *Bulletin of the Royal College of Psychiatrists 10*, 306–308.

Littlewood, R. and Lipsedge, M. (1988) 'Psychiatric illness among British Afro-Caribbeans.' *British Medical Journal 296*, 950–951.

Lloyd, K. (1992) 'Ethnicity, primary care and non-psychotic disorders.' *International Review of Psychiatry 4*, 257–266.

Lloyd, K. (1993) 'Depression and anxiety among Afro-Caribbean general practice attenders in Britain.' *International Journal of Social Psychiatry 39*, 1–9.

Lloyd, K. and Moodley, P. (1992) 'Psychotropic medication and ethnicity: an inpatient survey.' *Social Psychiatry and Psychiatric Epidemiology 27*, 95–101.

London Association of Community Relations Councils (1988) *In a Critical Condition: A Survey of Equal Opportunities in Employment in London's Health Authorities*. London: LACRC.

MacCarthy, B. and Craissati, J. (1989) 'Ethnic differences in response to adversity: a community sample of Bangladeshis and their indigenous neighbours.' *Social Psychiatry and Psychiatric Epidemiology 24*, 196–201.

Marger, M. (1991) 'Race and ethnic relations: American and global perspectives.' Belmont, CA: Wadsworth.

Marmot, M.G., Adelstein, A.M. and Bulusu, L. (1984) *Immigrant Mortality in England and Wales 1970–78*. London: HMSO.

Mather, H.M. and Marjot, D.H. (1989) 'Alcohol-related admissions to a psychiatric hospital: a comparison of Asians and Europeans.' *British Journal of Addiction 84*, 327–329.

May, A. (1994) 'Still they don't rise.' *Health Service Journal*.

McCreadie, R.G., Leese, M., Tilak-Singh, D., Loftus, L., MacEwan, T. and Thornicroft, G. (1997) 'Nithsdale, Nunhead and Norwood: similarities and differences in prevalence of schizophrenia and utilisation of services in rural and urban areas.' *British Journal of Psychiatry 170*, 31–36.

McGee, P. (1992) *Teaching Transcultural Care: A Guide for Teachers of Nursing and Health Care*. London: Chapman and Hall.

McGovern, D. and Cope, R. (1987a) 'First psychiatric admission rates of first and second generation Afro-Caribbeans.' *Social Psychiatry 22*, 139–149.

McGovern, D. and Cope, R. (1987b) 'The compulsory detention of males of different ethnic groups with special reference to offender patients.' *British Journal of Psychiatry 150*, 505–512.

McGovern, D. and Cope, R. (1991) 'Second generation Afro-Caribbeans and young whites with a first admission diagnosis of schizophrenia.' *Social Psychiatry and Psychiatric Epidemiology 26*, 95–99.

McGovern, D., Hemmings, P., Cope, R. and Lowerson, A. (1994) 'Long term follow-up of young Afro-Caribbean Britons and white Britons with a first admission diagnosis of schizophrenia.' *Social Psychiatry and Psychiatric Epidemiology 29*, 8–19.

McIver, S. (1994) *Obtaining the Views of Black Users of Health Services*. London: King's Fund.

McKeigue, P.M. and Karmi, G. (1993) 'Alcohol consumption and alcohol related problems in Afro-Caribbeans and South Asians in the United Kingdom.' *Alcohol and Alcoholism 28*, 1–10.

McKenzie, K., Os, J.V., Fahy, T., Jones, P., Harvey, I., Toone, B. and Murray, R. (1995) 'Psychosis with good prognosis in Afro-Caribbean people now living in the United Kingdom.' *British Medical Journal 311*, 1325–1328.

Mehtonen, O.P., Aranko, K., Malkonez, L. and Vapaatalo, H. (1991) 'Survey of sudden death associated with the use of antipsychotic or antidepressant drugs: 49 cases in Finland.' *Acta Psychiatrica Scandinavia 84*, 58–64.

Melzer, H., Cil, B. and Petticrew, M. (1994) *The Prevalence of Psychiatric Morbidity Among Adults Aged 16–64, Living in Private Households, in Great Britain.* ONS Surveys of Psychiatric Morbidity in Great Britain. Bulletin no.1. London: Social Survey Division, Office for National Statistics.

Mental Health Act (1983) London: HMSO.

Mental Health Act Commission (1989) *Third Biennial Report 1987–1989.* London: HMSO.

Mental Health Act Commission (1991) *Fourth Biennial Report 1989–1991.* London: HMSO.

Mental Health Act Commission (1995) *Sixth Biennial Report 1993–1995.* London: HMSO.

Mental Health Act Commission (1997) *Seventh Biennial Report 1995–1997.* London: HMSO.

Mental Health Act Commission (1999) *Eighth Biennial Report 1997–1999.* London: HMSO.

Mercer, K. (1984) 'Black communities' experience of psychiatric services.' *International Journal of Social Psychiatry 30,* 22–27.

Merrill, J. and Owens, J. (1986) 'Ethnic differences in self-poisoning: a comparison of Asian and white groups.' *British Journal of Psychiatry 148,* 708–712.

Merril, J. and Owens, J. (1987) 'Ethnic differences in self-poisoning: a comparison of West Indian and white groups.' *British Journal of Psychiatry 150,* 765–768.

MIND (1993) *Policy on Black and Minority Ethnic People and Mental Health.* London: MIND.

Mohan, D., Murray, K. Taylor, P. and Steed, P. (1997) 'Developments in the use of regional secure unit beds over a 12-year period.' *Journal of Forensic Psychiatry 8,* 2, 321–335.

Moodley, P. and Perkins, R.E. (1991) 'Routes to psychiatric inpatient care in an Inner London borough.' *Social Psychiatry and Psychiatric Epidemiology 26,* 47–51.

Moodley, P. and Thornicroft, G. (1988) 'Ethnic group and compulsory detention.' *Medicine, Science and the Law 28,* 324–328.

Morel, B.A. (1852) *Traite des Mentales.* Paris: Masson. Cited by Gottesman (1991).

Much, N. and Mahapatra, M. (1995) 'Constructing divinity.' In R. Harre and P. Stearns (eds) *Discursive Psychology in Practice.* London and Thousand Oaks, CA: Sage.

Mumford, B., Whitehouse, A.M. and Platts, M. (1991) 'Sociocultural correlates of eating disorders among Asian schoolgirls in Bradford.' *British Journal of Psychiatry 158,* 222–228.

Murphy, E. (1991) *After the Asylums.* London: Faber and Faber.

Murray, C. and Herrnstein, R. (1994) *The Bell Curve: Intelligence and Class Structure in American Life.* London: Free Press.

National Association of Health Authorities (1988) *Action Not Words, A Strategy to Improve Health Services for Black and Minority Ethnic Groups.* London: NAHA.

Nazroo, J.Y. (1997) *Ethnicity and Mental Health: Findings from a Community Survey.* London: Policy Studies Institute.

Neeleman, J., Jones, P., Van Os J. and Murray, R.M. (1996) Parasuicide in Camberwell: ethnic differences. *Social Psychiatry and Psychiatric Epidemiology 31*, 284–287.

Neeleman, J., Mak, V. and Wessely, S. (1997) 'Suicide by age, ethnic group, Coroner's verdict and country of birth. A three year survey in Inner London.' *British Journal of Psychiatry 171*, 436–467.

NHS and Community Care Act (1990). London: HMSO.

NHS Executive (1998) *A First Class Service – Quality in the new NHS*. London: NHSE.

NHS Executive Mental Health Task Force (1994) *Black Mental Health – A Dialogue for Change*. London: Department of Health.

Nichter, M. (1981) 'Idioms of distress: alternatives in the expression of psychosocial distress. A case study from South India.' *Culture, Medicine and Psychiatry 5*, 5–24.

Noble, P. and Rodgers, S. (1989) 'Violence by psychiatric inpatients.' *British Journal of Psychiatry 155*, 384–390.

Oberg, K. (1954) *Culture Shock*. Indianapolis: Bobbs-Merrill.

Observer (1999) Cabinet Office Advertisement, 12 September.

O'Callaghan, E., Sham, P., Takei, N., Glover, G. and Murray, R.M. (1991) 'Schizophrenia after prenatal exposure to 1957 A2 influenza epidemic.' *Lancet 337*, 1248–1250.

Odell, S.M., Surtees, P.G., Wainwright, N.W.J., Commander, M.J. and Sashidharan, S.P. (1997) 'Determinants of general practitioner recognition of psychological problems in a multi-ethnic inner-city health district.' *British Journal of Psychiatry 171*, 537–541.

Office for National Statistics (1995) *The Prevalence of Psychiatric Morbidity Among Adults Aged 16–64, Living in Private Households, in Great Britain*. ONS Surveys of Psychiatric Morbidity in Great Britain, Report 1. London: HMSO.

Office for National Statistics (1997a) *Key Data, 1997/8*. London: HMSO.

Office for National Statistics (1997b) *Regional Trends 32*. London: HMSO.

Office for National Statistics (1998) *Social Trends 28*. London: HMSO.

Ouseley, H. (1998) 'Missing Link.' *Nursing Standard 13*, 3.

Owen, M.J., Lewis, S.W. and Murray, R.M. (1988) 'Obstetric complications and schizophrenia: a computerised tomographic study.' *Psychological Medicine 18*, 331–339.

Owens, D., Harrison, G. and Boot, D. (1991) 'Ethnic factors in voluntary and compulsory admissions.' *Psychological Medicine 21*, 185–196.

Parkman, S., Davies, S., Leese, M., Phelan, M. and Thornicroft, G. (1997) 'Ethnic differences in satisfaction with mental health services among representative people with psychosis in South London: PRiSM Study 4.' *British Journal of Psychiatry 171* (Supplement 3), 260–264.

Peay, J. (1989) *Tribunals on Trial: Study of Decision Making under the Mental Health Act 1983*. Oxford: Clarendon Press.

Perera, R., Owens, D.G.C. and Johnstone, E.C. (1991) 'Ethnic aspects: a comparison of three matched groups.' *British Journal of Psychiatry 159* (Supplement 13), 40–42.

Persaud, A., Hanmore, G., Nagi, A. and Banga, P. (1998) *No, There's No Problem Here.* London: Department of Health and Wiltshire Health Authority.

Pfeffer, N. (1998) 'Theories of race, ethnicity and culture.' *British Medical Journal 317,* 1381–1384.

Pick, D. (1989) *Faces of Degeneration. A European Disorder, c.1848–c.1918.* Cambridge: Cambridge University Press.

Pilowsky, L.S., Ring, H., Shine, P.J., Battersby, M. and Lader, M. (1992) 'Rapid Tranquilisation: A Survey of Emergency Prescribing in a General Psychiatric Hospital.' *British Journal of Psychiatry 160,* 831–835.

Ponteroto, J.G. (1991) 'The nature of prejudice revisited: Implications for counselling intervention.' *Journal of Counselling and Development 70,* 216–224.

Ponteroto, J.G. and Pedersen, P.B. (1993) *Preventing Prejudice.* Newbury Park, California: Sage.

Prins, H., Blacker-Holst, T., Francis, E. and Keitch, I. (1993) *Report of the Committee of Inquiry into the Death in Broadmoor Hospital of Orville Blackwood and a Review of the Deaths of Two Other Afro-Caribbean Patients. Big, Black and Dangerous.* London: Special Hospitals Service Authority.

Prosser, D. (1996) 'Suicides by burning in England and Wales.' *British Journal of Psychiatry 168,* 175–182.

Qureshi, B. (1994) *Transcultural Medicine.* London: Kluwer Academic Publishers.

Race Relations Act (1976). London: HMSO.

Rack, P. (1982) *Race, Culture and Mental Disorder.* London: Tavistock.

Raleigh, V.S. (1996) 'Suicide patterns and trends in people of Indian subcontinent and Caribbean origin in England and Wales.' *Ethnicity and Health 1,* 55–63.

Raleigh, V.S. and Balarajan, R. (1992) 'Suicide and self-burning among Indians and West Indians in England and Wales.' *British Journal of Psychiatry 161,* 365–368.

Raleigh, V.S., Bulusu, L. and Balarajan, R. (1990) 'Suicides among immigrants from the Indian subcontinent.' *British Journal of Psychiatry 156,* 46–50.

Raleigh, V.S., Kiri, V. and Balarajan, R. (1996) 'Variation in Mortality.' *Health Trends 28,* 4.

Reich, W. (1991) 'Psychiatric diagnosis as an ethical problem.' In S. Bloch and P. Chodoff (eds) *Psychiatric Ethics.* Oxford: Oxford University Press.

Reiss, D., Grubin, D. and Meux, C. (1996) '"Young psychopaths" in special hospitals: Treatment and outcome.' *British Journal of Psychiatry 168,* 99–104.

Richie, J. (1964) 'Using an interpreter effectively.' *Nursing Outlook 12,* 27–29.

Ritchie, S. (1985) *Report to the Secretary of State for Social Services Concerning the Death of Mr Michael Martin at Broadmoor Hospital on 6th July 1984.* London: Department of Health and Social Security.

Rogers, A. and Faulkner, A. (1987) *A Place of Safety. MIND's Research Into Police Referrals to the Psychiatric Services.* London: MIND.

Royal College of Psychiatrists (1996) *Report of the Confidential Inquiry into Homicide and Suicide by Mentally Ill People, 1992–1996.* London: Department of Health/Royal College of Psychiatrists.

Rushton, J.P. (1990) 'Race differences, r/K theory, and a reply to Flynn.' *The Psychologist: Bulletin of the British Psychological Society 5*, 195–198.

Samuel, G. (1990) *Mind, Body, and Culture: Anthropology and the Biological Interface.* Cambridge: Cambridge University Press.

Sartorius, N., Jablensky, A., Korten, A., Ernberg, G., Anker, M., Cooper, J.E. and Day, R. (1986) 'Early manifestations and first-contact incidence of schizophrenia in different cultures.' *Psychological Medicine 16*, 909–928.

Sashidharan, S.P. (1993) 'Afro-Caribbeans and schizophrenia: the ethnic vulnerability hypothesis re-examined.' *International Review of Psychiatry 5*, 129–144.

Sashidharan, S.P. and Francis, E. (1993) 'Epidemiology, ethnicity and schizophrenia.' In W.I.U. Ahmad (ed) *'Race' and Health in Contemporary Britain.* Buckingham: Open University Press.

Scarman, Lord Justice (1981) *Report of the Inquiry into the Brixton Disorders, 10–12 April 1981.* Cm.8427. London: HMSO.

Secretary of State for Health (1997) *The New NHS: Modern and Dependable.* London: Department of Health.

Sen, B. and Williams, P. (1987) 'The extent and nature of depressive phenomena in primary health care: a study in Calcutta, India.' *British Journal of Psychiatry 151*, 486–493.

Sethi, B.B. (1986) 'Epidemiology of depression in India.' *Psychopathology 19*, Supplement 2, 26–36.

Shaikh, A. (1985) 'Cross-cultural comparison: psychiatric admission of Asian and indigenous patients in Leicestershire.' *International Journal of Social Psychiatry 31*, 3–11.

Shamasunder, C., Murthy, S.K., Prakash, O.M., Prabhakar, N. and Krishna, D.K.S. (1986) 'Psychiatric morbidity in a general practice in an Indian city.' *British Medical Journal 292*, 1713–1715.

Shetty, G. and Higgo, R. (1987) 'Compulsory detention of males of different ethnic groups.' *British Journal of Psychiatry 151*, 270.

Shubsachs, A.P.W., Huws, R.W., Close, A.A. and Larkin, E.P. (1995) 'Male 'Afro-Caribbean patients admitted to Rampton Hospital between 1977 and 1986 – a control study.' *Medicine, Science and Law 35*, 4, 336–346.

Simpson, G., Davis, J., Jefferson, J.W. and Perez-Cruet, J.F. (1988) *Sudden Death in Psychiatric Patients: The Role of Neuroleptic Drugs.* Task Force Report No.27. Washington DC: American Psychiatric Association.

Simpson, D. and Anderson, I. (1996) 'Rapid Tranquillisation: A Questionnaire survey of Practice.' *Psychiatric Bulletin 20*, 149–152.

Skellington, R. (1992) *Race in Britain Today.* London: Sage.

Smith, A.C. (1986) 'General and historical concepts in schizophrenia: Overview.' In A. Kerr and P. Swaith (eds) *Contemporary Issues in Schizophrenia.* London: Gaskell.

Snowden, L. and Cheung, F.K. (1990) 'Use of inpatient mental health services by members of ethnic minority groups.' *American Psychologist 45*, 347–355.

Social Exclusion Unit (1998) *Rough Sleeping.* Cmd 4008. London: HMSO.

Sone, K. (1992) 'Practice: mental illness. Unearthing hidden illness.' *Community Care*, 27 February.

Special Hospitals Service Authority (1989) *Report of the Inquiry into the Circumstances leading to the Death in Broadmoor Hospital of Mr Joseph Watts on 23 August 1988.* London: SHSA.

Special Hospitals Service Authority (1993) *The Use of Seclusion and the Management of Disturbed Behaviour within Special Hospitals.* London: SHSA.

Special Hospitals Service Authority (1995) *Service Strategies for Secure Care.* London: SHSA.

Sperber, D. (1975) *Rethinking Symbolism.* Cambridge: Cambridge University Press.

Stephen, S. (1997) 'Speaking Out.' *Nursing Times 93*, 5, January.

Stern, G., Cottrell, D. and Holmes, J. (1990) 'Patterns of attendance of child psychiatry outpatients with special reference to Asian families.' *British Journal of Psychiatry 156*, 384–387.

Sue, S., Fujino, D.C., Hu, L.T., Takeuchi. D.T. and Zane, N.W. (1991) 'Community mental health services for ethnic minority groups: a test of the cultural responsiveness hypothesis.' *Journal of Consulting and Clinical Psychology 59*, 533–540.

Sugarman, P. and Crauford, D. (1994) 'Schizophrenia in the Afro-Caribbean community.' *British Journal of Psychiatry 164*, 474–480.

Takei, N., Persaud, R., Woodruff, P., Brockington, I. and Murray, R.M. (1998) 'First episodes of psychosis in AfroCaribbean and white people. An 18 year follow-up population based study.' *British Journal of Psychiatry 172*, 147–154.

Taylor, P.J., Leese, M., Williams, D., Butwell, M., Daly, R. and Larkin, E. (1998) 'Mental disorder and violence: a special (high security) study.' *British Journal of Psychiatry 172*, 218–226.

Terman, L.M. (1916) *The Measurement of Intelligence.* Boston: Houghton.

The Times (1995) 'Link between schizophrenia and diabetes.' 13 April.

The Times (1998) 'Straw orders police to recruit minorities.' 20 October.

The Times (1998) 'Extra cash for schools to hire bilingual helpers.' 13 November.

The Times (1998) 21 November.

The Times (1998) 'Lawrence report to criticise nine officers.' 19 December.

The Times (1999) 'Patient wins "negro" row.' 2 September.

Thomas, A. and Sillen, S. (1972) *Racism and Psychiatry.* New York: Brunner Mazel.

Thomas, C.S., Stone, K., Osborn, M., Thomas, P.F. and Fisher, M. (1993) 'Psychiatric morbidity and compulsory admission among UK-born Europeans, Afro-Caribbeans and Asians in Central Manchester.' *British Journal of Psychiatry 163*, 91–99.

Tilki, M. (1998) 'The Irish connection.' *Housing Today*, 16 July.

Torkington, P. (1987) 'Sorry Wrong Colour.' *Nursing Times 83*, 24.

Turner, T.H., Ness, M.N. and Imison, C.T. (1992) 'Mentally disordered persons found in public places: diagnostic and social aspects of police referrals (Section 136).' *Psychological Medicine 22*, 765–774.

Turner, V. (1957) *Schism and Continuity in an African Religion: A Study of Ndembu Village Life.* Manchester: Manchester University Press.

Turner, V. (1980) *Celebration.* Washington, DC: Smithsonian Institute.

Turner, V. (1983) 'Body, brain and culture.' *Zygon 18,* 3, 221–245.

Van Os, J., Castle, D.J., Takei, N., Der, G. and Murray, R.M. (1996a) 'Psychotic illness in ethnic minorities: clarification from the 1991 Census.' *Psychological Medicine 26,* 203–208.

Van Os, J., Takei, N., Castle, D.J., Wessely, S., Der, G., MacDonald, A.M. and Murray, R.M. (1996b) 'The incidence of mania: time trends in relation to gender and ethnicity.' *Social Psychiatry and Psychiatric Epidemiology 31,* 129–136.

Vanzant, I. (1996) *The Spirit of a Man.* San Francisco: Harper.

Verges, F. (1996) 'To cure and to free: The Fanonian project of decolonized psychiatry.' In L.R. Gordon, T.D. Sharpley-Whiting and R.T. White (eds) *Fanon: A Critical Reader.* Oxford: Blackwell.

Verghese, A., John, J.K., Rajkumar, S., Richard, J., Sethi, B.B. and Trivedi, J.K. (1989) 'Factors associated with the course and outcome of schizophrenia in India.' *British Journal of Psychiatry 154,* 499–503.

Walker, N. and McCabe, S. (1973) *Crime and Insanity in England. Vol 2: New Solutions and New Problems.* Edinburgh: Edinburgh University Press.

Waxler, N. (1977) 'Is mental illness cured in traditional societies? A theoretical analysis.' *Culture, Medicine and Psychiatry 1,* 233–253.

Weatherall, J.G., Ledingham, J.G.G. and Warrell, D.A. (1996) *Oxford Textbook of Medicine.* 3rd edition. Oxford: Oxford University Press.

Weindling, P. (1989) *Health, Race and German Politics Between National Unification and Nazism, 1870–1945.* Cambridge: Cambridge University Press.

Wessely, S., Castle, D., Der, G. and Murray, R. (1991) 'Schizophrenia and Afro-Caribbeans: a case-control study.' *British Journal of Psychiatry 159,* 795–801.

Wessely, S.C., Castle, D., Douglas, A.J. and Taylor, P.J. (1994) 'The criminal careers of incident cases of schizophrenia.' *Psychological Medicine 24,* 483–502.

Williams, R. and Hunt, K. (1997) 'Psychological distress among British South Asians: the contribution of stressful situations and subcultural differences in the West of Scotland Twenty-07 Study.' *Psychological Medicine 27,* 1173–1181.

Wilson, A. (1985) *Finding a Voice – Asian Women in Britain.* London: Virago.

Wilson, M. and MacCarthy, B. (1994) 'GP consultation as a factor in the low rate of mental health service use by Asians.' *Psychological Medicine 24,* 113–119.

Wing, M. (1991) 'Racism in nursing.' *Share Newsletter,* Issue 1, November.

World Health Organisation (1973) *Report of the International Pilot Study of Schizophrenia.* Geneva: World Health Organisation.

World Health Organisation (1979) *Schizophrenia: An International Follow-up Study.* London: Wiley.

Yates, M. and Craddock, E. (1998) 'Culturally sensitive care in a forensic setting.' *Nursing Times 94,* 26, 68–69.

Contributors

Annie Bartlett is a Senior Lecturer and Consultant in Forensic Psychiatry at St George's Hospital Medical School and Springfield Hospital. She is additionally qualified in Social Anthropology. Her research interests include theory applied to the practice of psychiatry, study of institutions and evaluation of health services with particular reference to gender, ethnicity and sexual orientation.

Nizar Boga was born in Zanzibar, Tanzania. He came to England in 1960 and has since studied Environmental Health and Municipal Administration. He has also obtained a degree in Law from London University. He was Chief Environmental Health and Consumer Services Officer with Haringey Council and for the past five years he has worked as an investigator in the Local Government Ombudsman's Office. For at least nine years he has been an Imam in a London mosque and the visiting Imam at Broadmoor Hospital for seven years.

P.Q. Deeley studied Theology and Religious Studies at Clare College, Cambridge, before starting medical training at Guy's and St Thomas'. In 1993 he delivered the Gresham lectures in Divinity in conjunction with Professor John Bowker on gene-culture coevolutionary theories of religion. In 1995 he visited the All India Institute of Medical Sciences in New Delhi and elicited illness narratives from relatives of in-patients on the neurology and psychiatry wards. He is currently a registrar in psychiatry at the Maudsley Hospital in London.

Elaine Elvey graduated in English with several postgraduate qualifications, including a teaching diploma in music. She is the Chief Executive Officer of the Afro-Caribbean Mental Health Association and in the past she has worked on several committees at the Royal College of Psychiatrists. She is currently studying Law at the London School of Economics.

Suman Fernando, Sri Lankan by birth, was educated in Britain and worked as a psychiatrist in the NHS until he retired from full-time work in 1993. He was a member of the Mental Health Act Commission for nine years until October 1995 and chaired its National Standing Committee on Race and Culture. He is now involved in training, teaching and consultancy as Senior Lecturer in Mental Health at Tizard Centre, University of Kent at Canterbury. Also, he is involved in several organisations providing counselling and psychotherapy for black and Asian people.

Chandra Ghosh was educated in India and received her medical degree from Calcutta University. Since the early 1970s she has worked in the UK and gained a Diploma in Psychological Medicine and Membership of the Royal College of Psychiatrists. She was for ten years a Consultant Psychiatrist at Park Lane Hospital (later part of Ashworth Hospital) and subsequently Consultant Psychiatrist at Broadmoor Hospital. She is currently Medical Director for Pastoral Homes Ltd based at Hazlewood House, near Chesterfield.

Krishnan Gnanasekaran has been a Lecturer, Senior Lecturer, External Examiner, Researcher and Practitioner in both higher academic institutions and varied practice settings. He is currently Associate Director of Forensic Psychiatric Nursing Practice at Broadmoor Hospital.

Harvey Gordon has been a Consultant Forensic Psychiatrist at Broadmoor Hospital for 15 years. He is also clinical tutor in the Oxford region. He has a range of interests within forensic psychiatry, including ethnicity and religion.

Stan Grant is a qualified counselling psychotherapist working at Broadmoor Hospital with black men. He also has his own private practice in London. He is an independent trainer and facilitator with 14 years experience mainly in the public and voluntary sectors. His skills cover a broad spectrum of human relations issues, particularly in the areas of diversity, equality, cross-cultural issues and group facilitation and interpersonal dynamics.

Jayne Hayes completed her nurse training in 1988. Since then she has worked as a Ward Manager, a Practice Development Nurse and a Lecturer in both forensic and acute mental health environments. She is currently a Senior Nurse in a medium secure environment.

Chinyere Inyama is a solicitor running his own practice in central London with a Legal Aid Board Franchise in mental health and crime. Having obtained a BSc in Biochemistry and Pharmacology and an MSc in Experimental Pathology he worked for several years in medical research at the Royal Postgraduate Medical School before becoming a solicitor. Chinyere is a Law Society Mental Health Review Tribunal Panel interviewer, Mental Health Act Commissioner and member of MIND's Mental Health Act Working Group. He is currently undertaking PhD studies in the Philosophy and Ethics of Mental Health at the University of Warwick and has a special interest in the issues relating to ethnic minority patients in the mental health system.

Charles Kaye is a graduate of Manchester University where he studied English and American literature. After graduating, he joined the training scheme for hospital administrators organised by the King's Fund. After a number of posts in and around London, he was appointed District Administrator and later District General Manager in North Hampshire in the late 1970s. In 1989 he became Chief Executive of the Special Hospitals Service Authority where he remained until that body was dissolved in 1996. He is a fellow of the Institute of Health Care Management and was awarded the OBE in 1996. He is currently engaged on consultancy in service development and in training.

Alia Khan graduated in professional social work. She has extensive experience in youth and community work, with a special focus on the Asian community. As an accredited counsellor Alia manages the ASRA project – a support group for Asian women with mental health problems. She currently works as a Care Manager/ Development Worker with Buckinghamshire Social Services and is also studying for a Masters Degree in Business Administration.

Tony Lingiah commenced his professional career as a nurse and later graduated with both first and higher degrees in Education. He has been a lecturer since 1979 and is currently Professional Development Advisor for the Broadmoor Hospital Authority. In that capacity he has developed the 'Working With Difference' training programme which won the 1998 Health Service Management Award.

Georgina Linton is currently a Commissioning Manager with the High Security Psychiatric Services Commissioning Board DOH/NHS Executive, with particular responsibility for Broadmoor and Rampton hospitals. She is a qualified nurse for people with learning disabilities and a registered psychiatric nurse. In 1983, she was appointed by the Secretary of State to the Mental Health Act Commission where, during her ten-year tenure, she chaired the Special Hospitals Panel which co-ordinates the MHAC activities across the three high security hospitals, was involved in the development of the Commission's race and culture policy and was appointed a member of the Commission's Central Policy Committee. She has also worked as a Development Officer with MIND and was the Director of MIND South East region from 1992–95. From 1994–96 she served as a Non-Executive Director of the Lewisham and Guys Mental Health NHS Trust and chaired the Trust's Complaints and Serious Incidents committee.

Jane Mackenzie commenced her professional career as a psychiatric nurse practitioner and later graduated with a higher degree in quality management. She has extensive experience as a clinician in forensic practice and currently leads the Quality and Audit Programme at Broadmoor Hospital Authority. She has recently joined the Health Advisory Service Standards Development Programme in a substantive role on the Mental Health Team.

Carol Morgan-Clark has been Clinical Effectiveness and Audit Manager at Broadmoor Hospital since 1995. Prior to this she was Clinical Audit Manager at the Hammersmith Hospitals NHS Trust, having started in the audit field in 1992. She studied for an Open University degree, and recently obtained an MSc in Evaluation of Clinical Practice at the University of Westminster.

Margaret Orr After qualifying house jobs in Glasgow, she began GP training in Greenock, spending part of her time at the only prison for women in Scotland. Contact with the prison continued while working in the local maternity hospital where prisoners were delivered of their babies. Over the next ten years she continued this contact while working as a psychiatric registrar in Ravenscraig Hospital, Greenock. She later became a senior registrar at the Wessex Regional Secure Unit at Knowle Hospital, Fareham. Following four years as a Prison Medical Officer at HMP Winchester, Margaret became a Consultant Forensic Psychiatrist at Broadmoor Hospital in 1988. Between 1992 and 1994 she acted as Director of Medical Services at Broadmoor and was fully appointed to that post for a further fifteen months.

Albert Persaud is a Public Health Specialist for Wiltshire Mental Health Authority. He leads the work that the Authority is currently doing on mental health and the health needs of people from ethnic minorities. Apart from his clinical background, he has worked closely with the Centre for Mental Health Services in Development and the King's Fund. Nationally, he is a member of the Mental Health Act Commission, whose work includes monitoring the treatment and care of patients detained under the Act. He is a Board Member for the National Depression Campaign (formerly known as the Defeat Depression Campaign) and the Long Term Medical Conditions Alliance. In addition, he is on the UK Advisory Group of the World Health Organisation, Nations for Mental Health Programme.

Veena Soni Raleigh is a Senior Lecturer at the University of Surrey, working primarily on a national programme of public health monitoring and health outcomes research funded by the Department of Health. She has a special interest in the health of ethnic minorities in Britain. For a number of years she worked for international agencies on health and population issues in India, and she currently serves as a consultant to the Department for International Development (formerly ODA).

Index